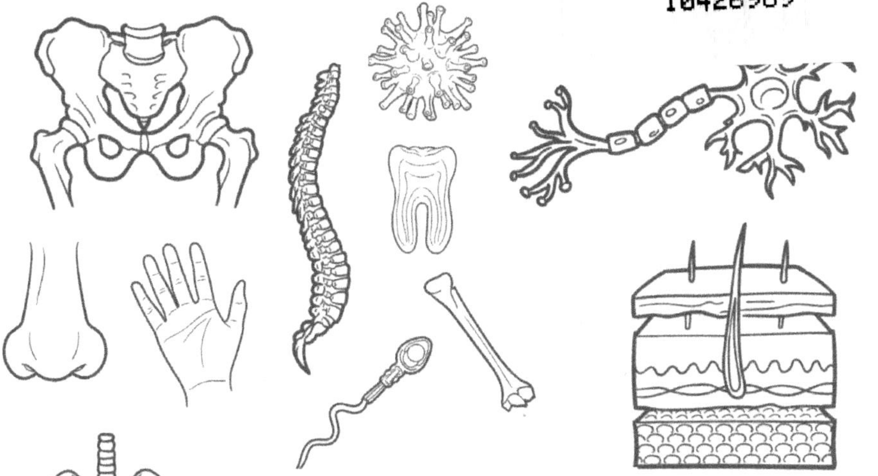

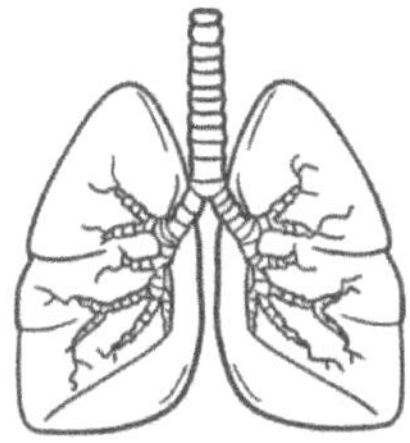

Ways
The Human Body
Can Go Wrong

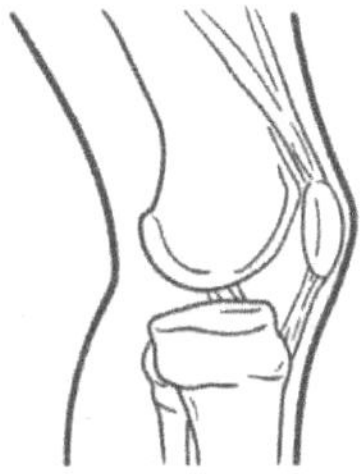

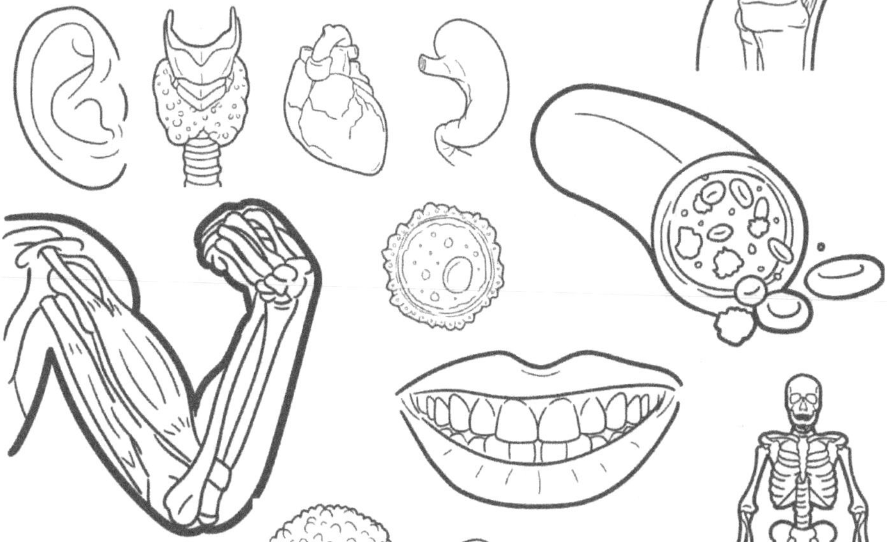

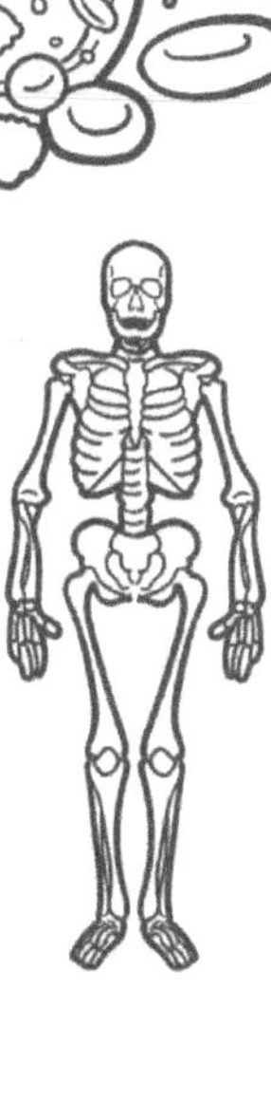

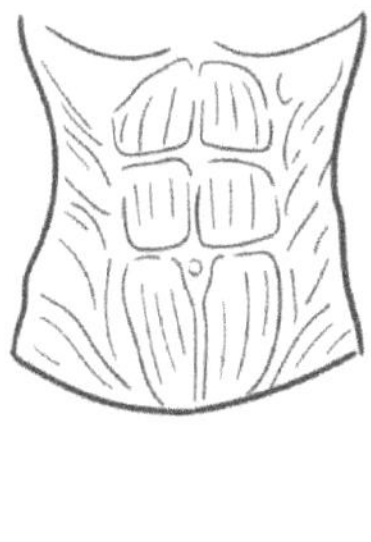

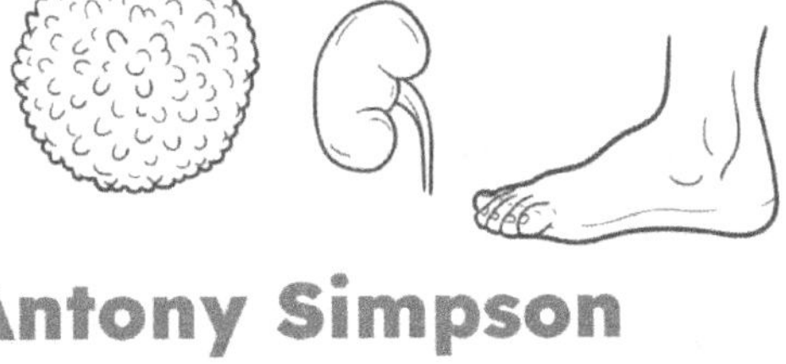

Antony Simpson

Antony Simpson's Website/Personal Blog: www.antonysimpson.com

Version 1.3

Other Books By The Author

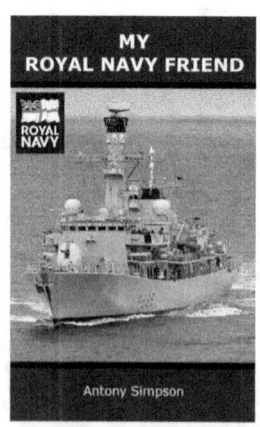

My Royal Navy Friend
My dear friend Roy decided to follow in his family's footsteps and enlist in the Royal Navy.

I wanted to maintain our friendship, to continue to support Roy, to make him laugh and to entertain him. So I came up with the idea of sending him a weekly email on random topics.

These emails were on a variety of topics, always being entertaining, sometimes being interesting, sometimes funny and occasionally being serious.

My Royal Navy Friend is a copy of these emails. In total, there are 52 emails. Dispersed throughout the book are also Royal Navy facts and stories.

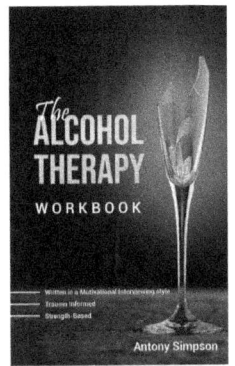

The Alcohol Therapy Workbook

This workbook has been designed for anyone that is struggling with alcohol or has struggled with alcohol in the past.

It is written in a Motivational Interviewing style, one of the key therapies used to support people with alcohol issues. It has been designed using a trauma-informed approach and is strength-based.

What you will find in this book is more than just worksheets about alcohol. You'll find all the tools someone needs to get into recovery from alcohol and stay there. It's a therapy-based book, not an alcohol-based book.

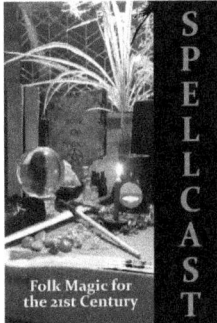

SpellCast - Folk Magic for the 21st Century (co-authored with Luna Hare)

SpellCast is a comprehensive compendium of spells, oils, charms and talismans. It is purely a book about magic, folk magic for the 21st century. The spells are ones that are tried and tested, with some that will stand the test of time.

In SpellCast you will read about the power of Instant Magic, of Banishment & Bindings, Blessings, Cleansing, Communication, Death, Employment, Finance & Money, Fertility, Friendship, Happiness & Joy, Health, Love & Relationships, Luck Magic, Protection, Transformative Magic and WishCraft. This book will change your life. Your life will be abundant in all meanings of the word.

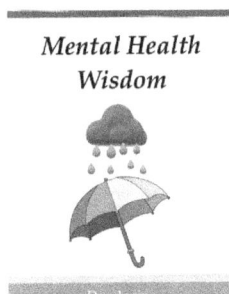

Mental Health Wisdom - Developing Understand & Empathy

This book contains everything that you need to know about mental health and mental illness.

Mental Health Wisdom is divided into three sections.

Understanding is section one and is all about the facts of mental health.

In section two, Empathy Through Lived Experience, the author shares his personal experience of mental illness.

Life Hacks is section three. It's all about self-care and quick and easy ways to improve your mental health, prevent mental illness or relapse of mental illness.

All available to buy in various formats internationally on Amazon.

If you enjoy this book please consider leaving a review on Amazon or Goodreads. Reviews are a great and free way to support the author.

DEADICATIONS

From the bottom of my heart and with eternal gratitude, I dedicate this book to:

Two incredible former Tutors of Childcare & Education at Wigan & Leigh College:
Linda Cunliffe & Brenda Nicholson.
Linda for her sage wisdom.
Brenda who gave me the best careers advice I ever got - 'Why don't you train to be a Nurse?'
Thank You.

Everyone who has ever taught me anything about the human body (and what can go wrong with it) including:
Patients & their Relatives
Colleagues from all Disciplines (Past and Present)
University Lecturers at UCLan
Family Members
Friends
Talkative Strangers on Buses.
Thank You.

For everyone who kindly agreed to review this book in its various draft forms and gave feedback.
Thank you, this book is ultimately much better thanks to your feedback.

To my Mum, Sarah, who should have been a Nurse.
Thank you for instilling confidence in me and for your continued love and support.

To My Brother Alex:
Your heart suddenly stopped when you were just 18 years old.
I miss you and think of you often.
It is and will always be devastating to me, how this outcome couldn't have been changed.

Contents

Healthcare: Clinical Excellence

To Conclude

Joke: Knock. Knock. Who's there? Doctor. Doctor Who.

Introduction

What amazes me, is just how many horrific ways the human body can go wrong.

As a Registered Nurse, I spent a number of years working in an Accident & Emergency (A&E) Department in a busy district general hospital. I was shocked by the number of ways the human body can go wrong on its own, without any lifestyle factors causing the malfunctions.

People who lived generally healthy lives were struck down by illness and diseases, through no fault of their own. Some conditions were curable, but most were not. For the latter, the only treatment is to manage the symptoms, prevent progression of the disease and prevent the damage caused for as long as possible.

I even got to experience this firsthand. At 21 years old, whilst a Student Nurse on placement in an A&E Department I became really unwell. I went to hospital, this time on the other side as a patient and was diagnosed with Diabetes (Type 1). Thanks immune system.

How can a complex organism, one with over 30 trillion cells, like the human body, fail in so many ways? I don't have the answer to this question.

But now I do know many horrific ways the human body can go wrong. That's what I share with you in this book.

Now, before I start. This book doesn't cover medical conditions that we cause by our own behaviour - such as overeating or not eating at all, smoking, drinking alcohol and taking drugs. It doesn't cover ultra rare diseases that affect very few people. If you want this sort of comprehensive book, go buy a medical encyclopaedia.

There is also humour spread throughout this book. This is because when suffering from a horrific body-go-wrong incident, people get to a point where they either laugh or cry. And I choose to laugh, always.

Let's start with dividing the human body into systems:

1. The Nervous System - This system consists of the brain, spinal cord and a network of nerves. I am reliably informed, by Brain Surgeons, that everyone has a brain, even those that come across like they're missing one.

2. The Sensory Organ System - This covers the eyes, ears, tongue and nose. Our sense of touch through our skin will be covered in the Integumentary System.

3. The Integumentary System - Consists of the skin (the body's largest organ), subcutaneous tissues, nails and hair.

4. The Skeletal System - The skeleton including: skull, rib cage, vertebrae, etc. It includes bone marrow, as well as cartilage, ligaments and tendons.

Joke: Why did the skeleton not go Trick-or-Treating at Halloween? He had no body to go with.

5. The Muscular System - This system includes all the muscles throughout the body.

6. The Lymphatic & Immune Systems - These include lymph nodes spread throughout the body, the spleen and the thymus. It includes white blood cells that float around in the Cardiovascular System.

7. The Respiratory System - This consists of the lungs and pharynx.

8. The Cardiovascular System - This consists of the heart, veins, arteries and blood.

9. The Endocrine System - This system is responsible for all those pesky hormones and includes the thyroid, the parathyroid and the glands (pituitary, pineal, and adrenal).

10. The Gastrointestinal System - This system deals with input and output and includes: mouth, teeth, oesophagus, stomach, liver, gallbladder, intestines and bowel.

11. The Urinary System - The bladder and kidneys make up the urinary system.

12. The Male Reproductive System - This is made up of the penis, testicles, prostate and sperm cells.

13. The Female Reproductive System - Much more complex than its male counterpart consists of the breasts, ovaries, fallopian tubes, womb and ovum cells.

14. System Wide Wrongs - This is basically any condition or disease that affects more than one system in the body; or where I couldn't squeeze it into any other chapter.

I have used these systems as chapter titles and we'll work through them together.

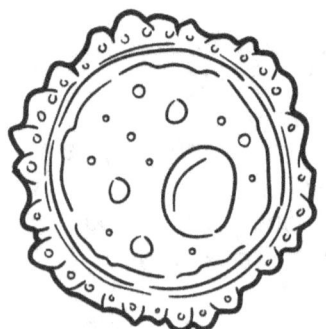

A human cell.

The final section of the book - Healthcare: Clinical Excellence contains a number of Appendices that give vital knowledge for Healthcare Professionals. This section of the book is an opportunity to learn from my experience as a Registered Nurse who has worked in a wide range of settings including A&E Departments.

Chapter 1 - The Nervous System

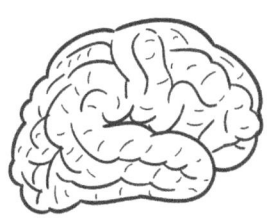

The Brain.

The brain is the boss of everything. It tells the heart to beat and the lungs to breathe. It also controls other countless involuntary processes.

The brain is responsible for our thoughts and feelings. It enables speech, eating, and exercise. It causes pain to tell us that something is wrong. It does everything. But the brain can go wrong in so many ways.

There is a distinction in modern medicine between physical and mental illness. But let us be clear: **mental illness is physical illness.** Mental illnesses are caused by neurons (brain cells) not working as they should.

Brain scans are becoming more common and we are learning that different areas of the brain are active and inactive in mental health conditions such as anxiety, bipolar, depression, obsessive compulsive disorder (OCD), schizophrenia and personality disorders. That being written, our understanding of the brain and how it functions is extremely limited.

Anxiety can be an acute or chronic condition. It is often described as uncontrollable worrying and feelings of dread. It isn't rational and can be triggered at any time. Even by something an individual has done a million times before without any anxiety. In severe cases it can be debilitating, affecting activities of daily living and causing panic attacks.

When we weren't at the top of the food chain, a bit of anxiety kept us alert to potential predators. But these days it seems to cause more harm than good. Anxiety causes more than just worry and dread, it causes physical symptoms including: sweating, increased heart rate, hot flushes and nausea.

Treatments for anxiety include anti-anxiety medication such as Citalopram and psychosocial therapies such as counselling and cognitive behavioural therapy (CBT).

Depression is a persistent low mood for a significant period of time. A person with depression will experience a wide range of emotions including: sadness, hopelessness, unhappiness and despair. Physical symptoms include exhaustion, difficulty sleeping, difficulty concentrating and short term memory loss. Depression can be triggered by life events or without any obvious trigger.

Treatments for depression include antidepressant medications and psychosocial therapies such as counselling or CBT.

Obsessive Compulsive Disorder (OCD) is a condition in which people with it have repetitive thoughts or behaviours. There is no cure for this illness, but people with OCD can learn to manage their symptoms through CBT. Sometimes, antidepressants are also used.

Bipolar is a mood disorder characterised by significant changes in mood, sometimes without any discernible trigger. The cause of bipolar is unknown and there is no cure. People with bipolar have episodes of high (or manic) mood (often where they become psychotic - losing touch with reality), episodes of low (severe depression) mood and episodes of feeling okay or numb, where they feel nothing.

Treatments for bipolar include a wide range of medications including antidepressants and antipsychotic mood stabilisers. Sometimes, counselling and CBT can be useful for helping a person with bipolar to cope with the mood states.

Schizophrenia is a severe mental illness. Symptoms include hallucinations, delusions, loss of touch with reality (medical term: psychosis) and being unable to complete activities of daily living. The exact cause of schizophrenia is unknown. There is no cure for schizophrenia. Treatment includes a range of antipsychotic medications and CBT.

Personality Disorders is an umbrella term to describe a range of disorders where the brain operates differently. People with a personality disorder think, feel and often behave very differently than the general population. The cause of personality disorders are unknown and there are no cures for personality disorders.

The specific type of Personality Disorder depends on the symptoms a person experiences. Medications (including antidepressants and antipsychotics), along with talking therapies (counselling, CBT and other psychosocial interventions) are used to manage the symptoms. However there is evidence suggesting that these are less effective than in people with other mental health illnesses.

People with Personality Disorder are at a significant risk of harm from themselves. Sadly, people with personality disorder often take their own life either intentionally or accidentally before the age of 40 years old.

Attention Deficit Hyperactivity Disorder (ADHD) is a neurological condition where the brain is structured differently to that of other people. The exact cause of ADHD is unknown, but sometimes it runs in families suggesting a genetic link. Symptoms of ADHD include impulsiveness, hyperactivity and difficulty concentrating. ADHD has a significant impact on activities of daily living and is usually picked up during childhood or when children start school.

If ADHD is left untreated it can have a significant impact on attainment and social relationships. ADHD is usually treated with medications, often stimulants which help an individual with ADHD focus.

Onto the 'physical' ways the brain can go wrong. The first is Acoustic Neuroma, it can also be called Vestibular Schwannoma. Acoustic neuroma (medical term) is a non-cancerous growth in the brain. The cause of these growths are unknown, they only grow on the nerves involved with hearing and balance. They don't spread to other parts of the body.

People with Acoustic Neuroma have problems with their hearing (including loss of hearing, hearing sounds coming from within the body and feeling the sensation of moving or spinning). A particularly large growth can also cause regular headaches, problems with vision (blurred or double vision), changes to voice, difficulty swallowing and numbness, weakness or pain to one side of the face. It can cause an unsteady gait, mimicking a drunk person's walk.

It is diagnosed through the presence of some of the symptoms above, with a Magnetic Resonance Imaging (MRI) scan of the brain. If the Acoustic Neuroma is small with a minimal impact on the person's life, a specialist doctor, known as a Neurologist, will monitor with regular MRI scans.

If a MRI scan shows a larger Acoustic Neuroma, surgery to have it removed is the only current treatment. Like all surgery, it is not risk-free. But it is the only treatment available. After surgery a repeat MRI scan will be undertaken. If there are any remains of the growth, it may be treated with radiotherapy.

The problem with Acoustic Neuroma is that they grow. The skull is a solid structure designed to protect the brain. So when the Acoustic Neuroma grows, it increases pressure on the brain.

This increased pressure, along with a build-up of fluid on the brain, can cause the brain stem, located in a little hole at the bottom centre of the skull, to get crushed. The brain stem sends messages to the heart to beat and the lungs to breathe. If it gets crushed it would be unable to send these messages and the body would cease to function, resulting in death.

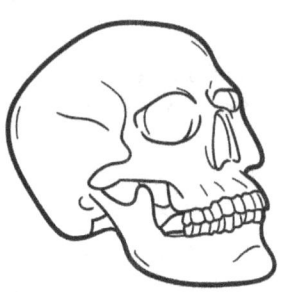

The Skull.

Even after going through surgery and radiotherapy a person with Acoustic Neuroma will need to continue regular MRI scans, as the growth in some cases returns.

The second is dementia. Dementia is split into a number of different types. But the symptoms are generally the same: changes to personality, short or long term memory loss, confabulation and confusion. Currently there are no cures for dementia, however treatments aim to slow the deterioration of the mind.

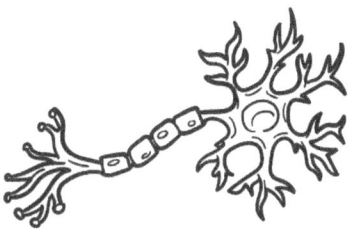

A neuron (brain cell).

In Epilepsy, neurons of the brain misfire causing seizures. These seizures vary massively from individual to individual, ranging from vacant episodes to grand mal seizures. Epilepsy is usually a lifelong condition and requires treatment from Neurologists and includes anti-epileptic medicines and sometimes a ketogenic diet.

Febrile Seizures (or Febrile Convulsions) occur in babies or children. The baby or child has usually been unwell with a raised temperature. The exact cause of Febrile Seizures is unknown but it is theorised that it is to do with the brain failing to 'turn down' the temperature when fighting an infection. This is thought to be due to an immaturity in a baby's or child's brain.

A Note On: Raised Body Temperature & Infections
When the human body is contaminated with a bacterial or viral infection, the body raises its temperature. This does two things inside the body:
1. It makes it harder for bacteria and viruses to survive and multiply.
2. It stimulates the immune system to respond, so that

> white blood cells are released to fight the infection.

The good news is that Febrile Seizures resolve themselves and that future Febrile Seizures can be prevented by:
- ❖ Stripping the baby/child down to minimum clothing when they have a temperature.
- ❖ Giving regular cold fluids to the baby/child.
- ❖ Ensuring the environment isn't too warm.
- ❖ Giving medications to the baby/child that lower the temperature (e.g. Paracetamol & Ibuprofen).

Babies/children grow out of Febrile Seizures as they get older. By around 7 years old, children are no longer at risk of Febrile Seizures.

A stroke is a life threatening condition which is caused when a blood clot forms or blood vessel bursts in the brain. It causes a limited or no supply of oxygenated blood to some neurons in the brain. The symptoms of a stroke are best remembered by FAST:
- → **F**ace - Maybe drooped. Someone having a stroke may also be unable to smile.
- → **A**rms - Someone having a stroke will struggle lifting up their arms and holding them there.
- → **S**peech - Their speech may be slurred or they may not be able to speak at all.
- → **T**ime - Time to call 999. The faster the treatment, the better the long term outcome.

There's also such a thing as a mini-stroke. The same symptoms apply, but are likely to be less severe. It's important to get mini-strokes treated, as they can lead to full strokes later on. Medications are generally used to treat strokes and mini-strokes. Occasionally surgery is required.

A Note On: Acute & Chronic Pain
Both acute (sudden onset) and chronic (long term) pain are the body's response to injury or damage. Pain is experienced thanks to sensory receptors (Nociceptors), which send messages through the nervous system to the brain. Pain is a very personal

experience and different individuals have different tolerance levels when it comes to pain.

Some diseases cause pain, as do some of the consequences of these conditions. Sometimes the source of pain can be easily identified. Whereas other times it can be difficult to identify the exact cause of pain.

Currently in the UK there are concerns about the numbers of people developing addiction/dependency to painkillers. This has led to a number of changes in the prescribing and dispensing of stronger painkillers. Due to the subjective nature of pain, sometimes medical professions can over or under prescribe in their aim of achieving effective pain management.

In my very personal experience of suffering with chronic pain recently, the doctors I've seen at my GP Surgery have under prescribed. This has left me at times in immense pain. I've broken down in tears in front of them to show my pain. I understand that doctors should always give the minimum amount of medications required to get the desired effects (as this reduces the chances of side effects), but it feels like they are not using the World Health Organization's (WHO) (1986) pain management ladder.

Charcot-Marie-Tooth Disease (CMT) is a number of conditions that damage Peripheral Nerves. The peripheral nerves are any nerves outside of the brain and spinal cord. They are genetic conditions that are inherited from their biological parents.

Symptoms can include muscle weakness to the hands, feet, ankles and legs, a way of walking that appears awkward and numbness to hands, arms and feet. Joint and nerve pain may also be present. Symptoms can begin to present at any age.

There are no cures for CMT and it is progressive, meaning it gets worse as time progresses. Treatments aim to keep individuals with CMT conditions as mobile and independent for as long as possible.

They include physiotherapy, occupational therapy and aids to assist with activities of daily living. A range of medications may be prescribed, along with surgery.

Counselling and CBT can help people with CMT to deal with their thoughts, frustrations and difficult emotions that may be triggered by their physical limitations as the disease progresses.

The brain has a blood-brain barrier (BBB) that is supposed to protect the brain from harmful organisms. Unfortunately it isn't always as effective as it should be. The BBB can become infected by both bacterial and viral Meningitis.

When this happens the BBB can become compromised and let the infection pass through to the brain. Meningitis can then damage the brain, sometimes permanently and in rare cases (usually where there is a significant delay in seeking medical treatment) can result in death.

Symptoms of Meningitis include a temperature of more than 37.5°C, confusion, headache, sometimes (but not always) a rash, a stiff neck, aches and pains, being sensitive to light, difficulty breathing or shortness of breath, having a reduced level of consciousness (late symptom) and seizures (late symptom).

Treatments for Meningitis include vaccinations to prevent Meningitis caused by certain bacterias, intravenous (injection into a vein) antibiotics in the case of bacterial Meningitis, intravenous fluids to prevent dehydration, antiviral medications for viral Meningitis, steroids to reduce swelling and inflammation and oxygen if short of breath.

Neurogenic Shock
Any type of shock in the human body is pre-terminal and likely to be treated in the Resuscitation section of an A&E Department.

Shock is where the body is not able to supply all the organs with enough blood. In shock, the human body rapidly deteriorates and can result in requiring Cardiopulmonary Resuscitation (CPR). Sadly around 20% of people who go into shock will die.

There are different types of shock, all of which shall be written about in the relevant chapters of this book. It is essential to understand that in shock the body focuses on supplying blood to the brain and the heart, to try and keep going for as long as possible.

Neurogenic shock is usually caused by damage to the nervous system (brain or nerves in the spine). The most common cause of Neurogenic shock is due to a spinal cord injury or trauma.

Cerebral palsy is an umbrella term for a number of conditions that affect a child before, during or shortly after birth. These conditions have in common that they affect movement and coordination. They are not usually spotted at birth but soon afterwards.

Causes of cerebral palsy include an infection in pregnancy, loss of blood supply to the unborn child's brain during pregnancy, stroke to unborn child, injury or trauma to unborn child, child being starved of oxygen during the birth, meningitis in the infant (see above) and low blood sugar (medical term: hypoglycemia) of infant at birth.

The risk of cerebral palsy is increased in premature babies, babies of a low birth weight, multiple pregnancies (such as twins or triplets) and alcohol/drug use during pregnancy.

Symptoms of cerebral palsy include:
* An infant being too stiff or floppy.
* Weak arms or legs.
* Developmental delay.
* Clumsy movements and poor hand-eye coordination.
* Delayed walking and then walking on tiptoes.
* Problems swallowing, learning disabilities, speaking problems and vision problems.

There is no cure for cerebral palsy, only treatments. Treatments depend on symptoms experienced but may include Occupational Therapy, Physiotherapy, Dietician input, Social Work input, Specialist Learning Disability Nurse input, Mental Health input and medications.

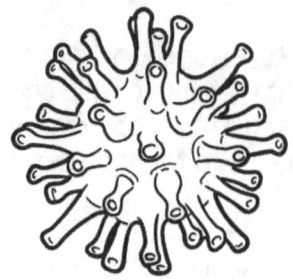

A virus cell.

Joke: Why was COVID-19 such a hit? Because it went viral.

Chapter 2 - The Sensory Organs System

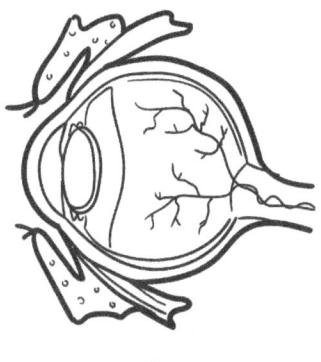

An Eye
(Internal View).

The eyes are the windows to the outside world. But they can malfunction in so many unexpected ways.

Even as children Amblyopia (Lazy Eye), Strabismus (Squints) and Colour Blindness are all eye-related problems.

For Amblyopia (Lazy Eye) treatment depends on the cause, but it is usually identified and treated before the age of 7-8 years old. Usually treatment involves glasses, by wearing an eye patch and sometimes eye drops.

These treatments are usually successful in treating a lazy eye, but do take time.

Strabismus (Squints) and Cataracts can cause a lazy eye to develop. Squints mostly occur in childhood, but can also occur in adults. The exact cause of a squint is usually unknown, but often comes along with other eye problems. The treatment for squints can include glasses, patches, eye exercises, injections into the affected eye and sometimes surgery.

Colour Blindness usually affects children, but weirdly can affect an adult at any point in their lives. There is thought to be a genetic link with colour blindness as it tends to run in families. But it can be caused by other eye or body conditions, a head injury, a stroke or certain medications as well. There is no cure or treatments for colour blindness, but people learn to live with the condition.

Age-related Macular Degeneration (AMD) is a rather misleading name, as it can start as early as 50 years old. The cause of AMD isn't fully known or understood, although some research suggests it might be linked to genetics or lifestyle factors such as being overweight or smoking.

AMD affects the vision either in one eye or both. It starts by distorting the vision in the centre of the eye and can lead to it turning into a black spot. The earlier the diagnosis the better, which is why people over 50 years old should have regular eye tests.

There are two main types of AMD - dry and wet. Dry AMD doesn't require treatment unless it becomes wet AMD and is caused by a build-up of a fatty substance behind one or both eyes.

Wet AMD is caused by the development of abnormal blood vessels behind one eye or both eyes. Sight deteriorates quickly. There is no cure for wet AMD but treatments include injection in the affected eyes and sometimes photodynamic therapy.

Unfortunately, current treatments for wet AMD only stop further deterioration of a person's eyesight, but doesn't reverse any of the damage already done.

Cataracts are clouding of the lens in the eyes that then affects vision. Cataracts usually affect both eyes, but in rare cases can affect just one. It is something that happens as humans get older, but we don't know why. Glasses are the initial treatment. When cataracts start to have a significant impact on vision, surgery is required to remove the cataracts.

Glaucoma is another eye condition that affects humans as they get older. It is caused by the optic nerve becoming damaged. The optic nerves connect the eyes to the brain so that sight is possible. Glaucoma usually affects both eyes at the same time, but not always. Glaucoma can take years to develop or come on quite suddenly.

When Glaucoma develops slowly it affects the edges of someone's vision very gradually, meaning that they often don't spot it themselves. This type of Glaucoma is usually spotted by an Optician during an eye test, which is why it is very important that older people have regular eye tests.

Sudden Glaucoma is usually accompanied by other systems including: severe pain to the eye or eyes affected, headaches, red eyes, tenderness around the eyes, blurred vision and feeling sick (medical term: Nausea) or vomiting.

The cause of Glaucoma is a failure in the ability of fluid to drain from the eye, causing increased pressure. There are several types of Glaucoma and the treatment depends on the type of Glaucoma. However, treatments include medications, eye drops, surgery and sometimes laser treatment.

Although treatments for Glaucoma have improved over time, there isn't currently a cure. Early identification and treatment is key to preventing further damage and slowing the progression of the disease.

Research studies vary massively in terms of the percentage of people with Glaucoma that go blind. But these research studies are often longitudinal because Glaucoma is so slow to progres. This means that people with Glaucoma may die of old age or other diseases before they go fully blind.

Refractive Errors, more commonly known as being short-sighted or long-sighted are another way the eyes can fail. They are characterised by the inability to focus clearly on either things far away (short-sighted) or things close (long-sighted). Instead of being clear, things are blurry.

The cause of Refractive Errors are unknown. But glasses or contact lenses can enable a person to see clearly despite Refractive Errors. Laser or Lens surgery can sometimes cure these conditions - although this is not guaranteed. Although the risk of laser surgery going wrong is pretty low, it is still a possibility.

Astigmatism is when someone's eyes are shaped like a rugby ball, rather than like a football. It is usually picked up by an Optician during an eye test and can cause blurry vision. It is treated the same way as Refractive Errors are.

Diabetic Retinopathy is a condition that affects the eyes due to a person with diabetes having high blood sugars over a prolonged period of time. For more details about Diabetes see 6 - The Lymphatic & Immune System (p48-52) chapter in this book.

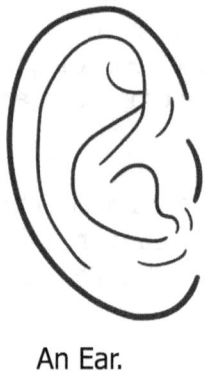

An Ear.

Ears are an important part of the human body. Not only do they help a person hear what's going on around them, they also assist with balance. They enable people to listen to the breakup songs of Taylor Swift.

Polyps are something you'll read about in various chapters of this book. Any sort of polyps are non-cancerous growths. They serve no purpose and usually cause pain and other symptoms.

Aural Polyps are growths outside the ear canal or in the middle ear. The cause of Aural Polyps is usually Cholesteatoma (see below), an infection causing inflammation in the ear, a traumatic injury to the ear, a foreign object stuck in the ear or Cancer within the ear. The most typical symptom is a bloody discharge from the affected ear, with or without pain. But other symptoms can include: hearing loss and feeling like the ear is permanently blocked.

Prior to treatment, identifying the cause of Aural Polyps is essential. In terms of the polyps themselves, surgery to remove them is the usual treatment. A Computed Tomography (CT) scan may be performed before the surgery. This CT scan assists the Surgeon in assessing the polyps for removal.

Antibiotics (both ear drops and/or oral) may be used if the cause is a bacterial infection or to prevent infection following surgery. Steroid medications may be prescribed to reduce inflammation and swelling caused by the polyps.

During the ear surgery to remove the polyps a biopsy is usually undertaken, especially if the cause of the polyps is unclear. Post operatively an individual with Aural Polyps will require time to recover before they are able to return to work and other activities of daily living.

Cholesteatoma is a particularly nasty ear condition where part of the eardrum collapses and this causes a collection of dead skin cells to build-up. It usually affects one ear. People can be born with Cholesteatoma but this is rare. Injury, infection or ear surgery (for other reasons) are thought to be the causes of Cholesteatoma.

Cholesteatoma is usually first identified due to symptoms which include a constant watery discharge from the affected ear, that may come and go. Sometimes this discharge may have a distinct smell, but not always. Some people get ear pain or discomfort, but not always. Another symptom is hearing loss in the affected ear. It is diagnosed by a medical assessment and CT scan.

It is really important that Cholesteatoma is treated, as it can lead to other complications if allowed to develop. These other complications include an ear infection (that can spread to the brain), an abscess on the brain, permanent hearing loss, damage to facial nerves, vertigo and tinnitus.

The treatment is surgery to remove Cholesteatoma with time to recover afterwards. In some cases, further surgery may be required to repair damaged parts of the ear. Although this second surgery is not always successful in repairing the damage that has been caused.

During the recovery period (which is around two weeks) it is advised that the ear is kept dry and that flying and strenuous activities are avoided. Unfortunately Cholesteatoma can reoccur, requiring further surgery and medications to treat it.

Deafness or hearing loss is a general term used to describe deterioration in someone's ability to hear. It is often gradual. It has a number of causes and is often treatable, with treatments that can sometimes improve a person's hearing. You can be born deaf, so it is important that children are taken for hearing tests from a young age.

Causes of deafness include: deafness caused by general ageing (treatable with hearing aids), ear infections (treatable with antibiotics), a build-up of earwax (treatable - see below), a perforated eardrum (treatable - see below) and Ménière's Disease (treatable - see below).

Joke: I fell out with Joe, my deaf friend, because he never listens.

Earwax can build-up causing difficulty in hearing in one or both ears. This is easily treated with ear drops or medical grade olive/almond oil available from a pharmacy. It is more often experienced by older people and we don't have an explanation for why some people struggle with earwax build-up and others don't. But the treatment is straightforward, can often be completed by an individual at home and should be painless.

A Perforated Eardrum is a hole in your eardrum. It is usually caused by an ear infection, injury to the ear, loud noise (either sudden or continual) or a change in pressure (such as when flying). Usually it affects one ear. Symptoms include hearing loss, pain, tinnitus, dizziness, itchiness and sometimes a discharge from the ear.

Perforated eardrums usually resolve on their own, but occasionally require medical attention to treat the underlying cause (e.g. antibiotics for a bacterial infection).

Ménière's Disease is a rare condition that can be difficult to diagnose due to the symptoms being similar to other ear conditions such as vertigo, tinnitus, pain, hearing loss, nausea (feeling sick) or vomiting and occasionally losing balance. The cause of Ménière's Disease is unknown and there isn't a cure. But treatments aim to improve symptoms and include medications to help manage symptoms and in some cases hearing aids.

A condition called Glue Ear is common in childhood, although can affect adults as well. It can sometimes clear up on its own in about three months without any medical treatment. Glue Ear is caused by the middle part of the ear canal filling with fluid.

The main symptom of Glue Ear is hearing loss. But other symptoms can include earache, tinnitus and difficulties with balance. Glue Ear can have an impact on a child's development, education and wellbeing. This is why it is important to get children's ears checked regularly, so that any symptoms can be spotted early on.

A treatment for Glue Ear is called Autoinflation and involves inflating a special balloon inside a child's nose, one nostril at a time. This helps the fluid in the ear to drain.

Another treatment is the surgical insertion of grommets. Grommets are tiny tubes inserted into one or both ears of a child, which keep their eardrums clear of fluid.

These grommets naturally fall out as a child continues to grow within 6-12 months. Grommets are so tiny that children and parents/carers very often never see the grommets as they fall out or after they have fallen out. On some occasions, some children might need to have grommets inserted more than once.

Grommets have an immediate impact, instantly improving a child's hearing. The surgery is very low risk and the operation is completed in a relatively short period of time in hospital. Children go home with their parents/carers the same day.

But as the children are put under general anaesthetic, I can't write that there aren't any risks. These should be explained to the parents/carers before the operation and informed consent should be obtained for the surgery.

To reassure any parents/carers reading this, what I can say is that the National Health Service (NHS) completes hundreds of thousands grommet operations on children per year (inserting millions of grommets). In all my years of practice as a Nurse, I have never experienced or heard of a case going wrong.

Otosclerosis is a condition characterised by loss of hearing, tinnitus and problems with balance. It is caused by Stapes bone in the ear fusing to other parts of the ear. It can affect one or both ears.

There is thought to be a genetic link with Otosclerosis, as you are much more likely to experience the condition if someone in your family has it. Here's a fun fact: the Stapes bone is the smallest bones in the human body.

Otosclerosis is generally diagnosed by CT scan and treatment is either by hearing aids or surgery. The surgical option involves replacing the Stapes bone with either a plastic or metal implant. The surgery is said to be extremely successful in terms of restoring hearing.

As the surgical option for Otosclerosis is carried out under general anaesthesia it is not without risk. But for many people when weighing up the potential benefits versus the potential risks, the benefits are more important than the risks.

Swimmer's Ear, known medically as Otitis Externa is a condition where the external ear canal gets swollen and inflamed. It can be caused by a bacterial or fungal infection, irritation or allergies.

It got its 'Swimmer's Ear' name because regularly getting water in the ears leaves them vulnerable to infections and inflammation. Wet ears can be itchy, causing a person to scratch and potentially cause a break in the skin in the ear canal. Water also makes the ear canal a moist environment, which is perfect for bacteria and fungi cells to multiply.

Tinnitus and Vertigo are more symptoms rather than conditions in themselves. That is not to minimise how severe these symptoms can be. Tinnitus is when someone hears sounds that don't come from an outside source. These sounds include buzzing, ringing, humming, hissing and throbbing.

Vertigo comes in episodes and is feeling like the world around you is spinning out of control. Vertigo episodes vary in intensity and length of time. Vertigo can last anywhere from from a few seconds to many days. Severe episodes of Vertigo have even been known to last months and are debilitating.

Vertigo can sometimes resolve itself without any treatment. But other times it requires medical attention to identify and treat the underlying cause triggering these Vertigo episodes.

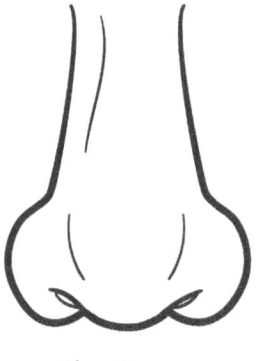

The Nose.

The nose enables us to smell dog foul at a hundred paces away, yet some people still manage to stand in it and have to spend time scraping it off their shoes.

The nose, like anything else in the body, can go wrong. This includes conditions such as Allergic Rhinitis, Chronic Rhinosinusitis, a Deviated Septum, a Perforated Septum and Nasal Polyps.

Allergic Rhinitis is a reaction to something the body has developed an allergy to such as dust, animals, grass or other stimuli. Symptoms include irritated nasal passages, sometimes with swelling, a runny nose, a blocked nose, watering eyes and an itchy nose/roof of mouth. Allergic Rhinitis affects can vary from very mild to very severe.

There is no cure for Allergic Rhinitis but it can be managed or treated. The best way to manage Allergic Rhinitis is to identify the environmental trigger and if possible remove it.

If this is not possible Allergic Rhinitis can be treated with antihistamine and decongestant medications. In severe cases of Allergic Rhinitis, a GP can prescribe stronger medications (including steroids) or may refer an individual to an Ear, Nose & Throat (ENT) Consultant.

Chronic Rhinosinusitis is swelling of the nasal passages lasting three months or longer. Symptoms also include nasal discharge, blocked nasal passages, nasal drip and a reduced sense of smell. It can sometimes be accompanied by a Deviated Septum, a Perforated Septum and Nasal Polyps (see below for details of these conditions), but not always. Sometimes the cause of Chronic Rhinosinusitis can be a nasal or sinus infection.

Cases of Chronic Rhinosinusitis should be referred to ENT Consultant. Treatments can include medications (steroids, antibiotics, antihistamines, nasal sprays) and sometimes surgery.

The Septum is the piece of cartilage that separates and forms the two nasal passages. In the case of a Deviated Septum the Septum either grows abnormally or is damaged by an accident or injury. Symptoms of a Deviated Septum are similar to those of Chronic Rhinosinusitis. Surgery is required to correct the deviation.

A Perforated Septum is when a hole develops in the Septum. This hole can have a number of causes including:

❖ Accident or injury to the Septum, including during previous surgical procedures to the nose or through excessive nose picking.

❖ Repeated nasal infections that eventually eat away at the Septum.

❖ Substance use taken into the body nasally such as cocaine or ketamine.

❖ Some very rare autoimmune conditions.

❖ Nasal cancer.

❖ Sometimes the cause is unknown.

A Perforated Septum has the same symptoms as Chronic Rhinosinusitis, but with some additional ones including pain (which can be severe), crusting in the nasal passages, a foul smell coming from within the nose and sometimes a whistling sound from the nose.

Surgery is required to fix a Perforated Septum. This is done by either placing a 'button' in the hole or placing ear/rib cartilage from the individual in the nose. Surgery is usually a day case with good results.

The cause of Nasal Polyps is unknown. Nasal Polyps are non-cancerous growths in the nose. Symptoms are the same as Chronic Rhinosinusitis. Nasal Polyps can be extremely painful. Steroid medications can reduce the size of the polyps, but surgery to remove them is usually required. The initial surgical results are effective and resolve the issue, but Nasal Polyps can return in some cases.

Ways the mouth, tongue and teeth can go wrong will be covered in chapter 10 - The Gastrointestinal System (p89-101).

Joke: Why are Health Professionals always calm?
Because they have a lot of patients.

Chapter 3 - The Integumentary System

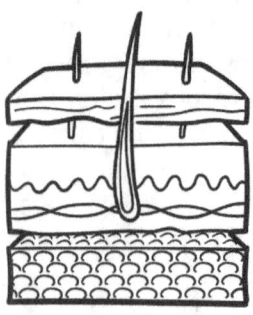

Layers of the Skin.

You wouldn't think much could go wrong with the skin, nails and hair on the human body. But you'd be wrong. Especially with the skin. I honestly thought the skin was there just to keep the organs on the inside of the body.

But with the skin you've got Psoriasis, Acne, Eczema, Vitiligo and Keratosis Pilaris. All conditions where the body gets it wrong.

Want to look like a snake shedding its skin? No problem, the human body has you covered with Psoriasis. Psoriasis causes your skin to develop red, very itchy, scaly patches. These patches usually appear on elbows, knees, scalp and lower back.

Acne or spots is another way the human body goes wrong. Acne is the result of too much oil on your skin, which blocks your pores and causes spots. What's most annoying about this body failing is that one of the main places people get acne is on their face. You know, the part of the body everyone sees and looks at.

Eczema causes the sufferer's skin to become itchy, dry and cracked. It is thought that food, certain skin products, the weather, hormones and stress can trigger an eczema episode. So basically, practically anything.

Psoriasis, Acne and Eczema are generally treated using a range of prescribed topical medications. Sometimes oral medications are prescribed and on rare occasions laser treatments can be used.

Vitiligo is a condition which causes light patches to appear on the skin due to a lack of melanin pigment. These lighter patches of skin can appear anywhere on the body but are more likely to occur on the face, hands and neck.

Vitiligo is a failing of the immune system and sadly not the only way your immune system doesn't work correctly. You'll discover other ways the immune system gets things wrong by reading this book.

Unfortunately the lighter patches of skin in Vitiligo are usually permanent. This can affect a person's self-esteem and confidence. There are some temporary treatments to make the patches of skin less noticeable, but they only work on a short term basis and don't stop the patches from increasing in size or new patches from developing.

Keratosis Pilaris is when small bumps appear on the skin. Sometimes the skin may also become rough and dry. These small bumps are painless but may be itchy. They usually appear on the bottom, thighs or arms, but like any skin condition can appear anywhere.

The cause of Keratosis Pilaris is too much keratin, a protein that makes up the outer layer of the skin. Treatments for this condition include a course of steroid creams applied topically to the affected areas or laser treatment. The treatments do help, but as they aren't a cure and Keratosis Pilaris can reappear.

Lichen Planus is a rash that not only affects the skin, but also the mouth, tongue and genitals. The cause is not known or fully understood. The rash is sometimes itchy, but not always. Doctors can prescribe medications for the rash and itchiness. The rash itself usually clears up after 9-18 months. What a long time to suffer with this disease.

Your nails are the most reliable part of the Integumentary System. Nothing usually goes wrong with finger or toe nails. Remarkably, they can even give an indication of long term medical conditions such as anaemia (iron deficiency), thyroid problems, diabetes and heart/lung/liver disease.

Alopecia is a medical term for hair loss on both males and females. Hair loss in males on the head is not considered a medical condition and usually runs in families, indicating some genetic link. Sometimes hair loss is temporary and sometimes it is permanent, it just depends on the cause.

Causes of hairloss include: genetics, illnesses, iron deficiency and treatments for cancer.

If temporary alopecia, the underlying disease should be treated and as time progresses the hair will grow back.

There are a couple of medications that can sometimes help, but they only work for as long as you keep taking them. Plus like all medications, there's always a risk of side effects. Immunotherapy, light treatments and a hair transplant are all alternative treatments for alopecia.

Another option is to wear a wig like Elton John. But whether a wig is made with synthetic or real hair, they always look like a wig, don't they?

Chapter 4 - The Skeletal System

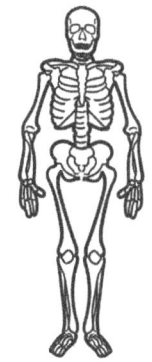

The skeletal system has a total of 206 bones. They vary in size, dependent upon function.

The skull and rib cage's function for example is to protect our brain and other vital organs (the heart & lungs).

Most bones have bone marrow inside of them, which is where red blood cells, white blood cells and

The Skeleton.

and platelets are created. For more information about blood cells see p68-69.

Despite how durable we often consider bones to be, there are actually quite a few malfunctions that can occur. Osteopenia is the first stage of Osteoporosis. Osteopenia is usually diagnosed through a scan on the bones. There are treatments and lifestyle changes that reduce the risk of Osteopenia becoming Osteoporosis; but they are not guaranteed to prevent Osteoporosis.

Osteoporosis is losing density in bones. A person with Osteoporosis is at greater risk of breaking bones (medical term: fractures) through falls and other accidents. In severe cases of Osteoporosis broken bones can be caused by normal everyday activities. For example, a cough or sneeze can result in a rib or spinal fracture.

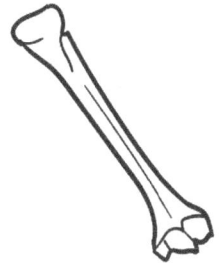

The exact cause of Osteopenia & Osteoporosis isn't known. It is normal for the body to lose some bone density as people age. But this doesn't explain why some people lose more bone density and more quickly than others.

It is useful to know things that increase the risk of developing Osteopenia & Osteoporosis. They are:

- ❖ Taking steroid medications for more than three months.
- ❖ A range of other medical conditions, particularly ones that cause inflammation and changes to hormone levels.
- ❖ Having someone in the family that's been diagnosed with Osteoporosis. This suggests that sometimes there are genetics playing a role.
- ❖ Having or previously had poor dietary intake, including eating disorders.
- ❖ Having a low Body Mass Index (BMI).
- ❖ Lack of exercise.
- ❖ High levels of alcohol use.
- ❖ Smoking.
- ❖ Specific to Females, Menopause increases the risk. Particularly if it's early onset. But the conditions don't just affect females.

The current thinking with Osteoporosis is that it is better to prevent it rather than treat it. There is no cure for Osteoporosis, but there are good treatments available.

Preventing Osteoporosis is about lowering risk. Regular exercise, taking vitamin supplements (including Calcium and Vitamin D), reducing or stopping alcohol/smoking can all help lower the risk. But these actions don't eliminate the risk completely.

Treatments for Osteoporosis involve medications to strengthen bones and taking Calcium and Vitamin D supplements. Treatment for broken bones include a bone scan in people 50 years old or older to screen for Osteoporosis, painkillers, sometimes a cast, recovery physiotherapy and occasionally surgery.

Osteomyelitis is a bacterial infection of the bone. It is caused by bacteria and easily treated with oral or intravenous (injections into the vein) antibiotics. Delays in seeking medical attention can result in complications such as the infection spreading, abscesses and worst case scenario can be life-threatening.

Paget's Disease of Bone is a condition caused by faulty bone modelling cells. There are two bone cells responsible for keeping bones healthy: osteoclasts and osteoblasts.

Osteoclasts bone cells are responsible for absorbing old cells that make up a bone.

Osteoblasts bone cells are responsible for producing new cells to replace the ones that the Osteoclasts absorb.

In Paget's Disease of Bone the Osteoclasts absorb bone cells much more quickly than they are supposed to. The Osteoblasts rush their production of bone cells to try to keep up, but the cells they produce are weaker than what they should be.

Paget's Disease of Bone is a common condition in the 50+ years old population. People who have a family history of Paget's Disease of Bone are at an increased risk of experiencing it themselves as they get older. This suggests a genetic link.

There isn't a cure for Paget's Disease of Bone. Treatments focus on symptom management. Symptoms of this condition include: pain in bones, changes to the shape of bones, an increased risk of fractures and in some cases no symptoms at all (in these cases it is discovered whilst undertaking tests and investigations for other diseases or conditions).

Treatments for Paget's Disease of Bone include medications, physiotherapy, occupational therapy and sometimes surgery.

Joke: What do you call a skeleton having a party? An Osteoblast.

Rickets were common at one time in the UK due to poor dietary intake. It occurred during childhood with the effects lasting into adulthood. Rickets are caused by a lack of Calcium and Vitamin D. Whenever I think of Rickets I think of bowed legs. But it has a range of symptoms including: pain, fragile bones that are more prone to fractures, deformity of bones, stunted growth and developmental delays.

It is easier to prevent rickets through good nutrition, rather than to treat the consequences of it. Treatments are Calcium and Vitamin D supplements, along with treatments to treat the consequences of the condition (i.e. painkillers, casts, etc. to treat fractures).

There are a few forms of genetic rickets. These have a genetic cause, but symptoms are the same as rickets. Treatments depend on the type of genetic rickets, But they are treatable. I'm not going into detail on these types of rickets as they are exceptionally rare.

Rickets is having a resurgence in the UK and is linked to increasing levels of health inequality and poverty.

Brittle Bone Disease, known by its medical name Osteogenesis Imperfecta, is a genetic disease without a cure. It affects the protein collagen which helps make bones strong. In someone with Brittle Bone Disease, their bodies might not make enough collagen, or it does make enough collagen but it is of poor quality.

Brittle Bone Disease is on a spectrum of severity. It is often characterised as mild, moderate or severe by doctors. In severe cases fractures to bones can occur without injury, mobility is impaired and fatigue is experienced. Quality of life could be significantly impacted.

Treatments for Brittle Bone Disease include: medications, Vitamin D supplements, physiotherapy, social worker support and immediate treatment of any fractures.

Osteonecrosis or Avascular Necrosis is when blood supply is cut off to the end of a bone. The blood supply being cut off results in death of bone cells. Usually the cause of Avascular Necrosis is never found. But once the blood supply is cut off and the cells have died it is not reversible or curable.

Avascular Necrosis causes the bone to change shape, can cause joint pain but sometimes there's no symptoms at all. It is usually diagnosed through an X-Ray. Treatment is usually to manage the joint pain and stiffness. So painkillers and anti-inflammatory medication and physiotherapy help. Very occasionally surgery may be required. Pain and joint stiffness can last for 12-18 months and should improve as time passes.

Fibrous Dysplasia is a genetic mutation, but it is not inherited from biological parents. The mutation develops in the womb. It is a condition that affects one or more bones. It causes affected bones to get stuck in the immature fibrous stage of development. This means that the affected bones are weak and can misshapen.

Fibrous Dysplasia is usually identified by its symptoms: swelling of the jaw, gaps between the teeth, possible unequal limb length (if bones in one leg are affected) and unexpected fractures. Fibrous Dysplasia is usually diagnosed through a variety of radiographic scans including X-Rays, CT scans and MRI scans.

Unfortunately there is no cure for Fibrous Dysplasia and treatments focus on symptom management.

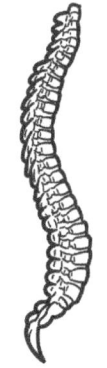

The Spine.

Scoliosis always reminds me of the film *Romy & Michelle's High School Reunion*. If you've never seen this film, it's a fantastic American comedy, starring Mira Sorvino & Lisa Kudrow (Phoebe from Friends).

Scoliosis is a spinal condition where the spine grows with a curvature or deviation from normal upright straightness. It is usually identified in childhood, although certain types of Scoliosis can affect adults. The cause of Scoliosis isn't known, but it is likely to be related to genetics as it tends to run in families.

Symptoms of Scoliosis are a visible curvature, an affected individual leaning to one side, a shoulder or hip sticking out on one side and clothes not fitting well.

Treatments depend on the age of the person but may include monitoring (to see if with time it resolves itself), a cast, possibly back exercises (as recommended by a health professional with expertise in Scoliosis), a back brace and sometimes surgery to straighten the spine. It is generally a painless condition, but in the case of it causing back pain - painkillers are prescribed.

The back cast or back brace can affect a person's ability to participate in some sports or physical activities, but only in the short term while it is in place. Back casts or back braces may also impact on a child's or adolescent's self-esteem.

By adulthood Scoliosis has usually resolved, if treated. The outlook for a child with Scoliosis is extremely positive. The life expectancy is that of a person of the same gender who didn't have Scoliosis. They can fully participate in life once the Scoliosis has resolved and looking at a person who had Scoliosis as a child, you wouldn't know that they had it as an adult.

On rare occasions Scoliosis can be caused by an underlying condition such as the spine not developing correctly in the womb or nerve/muscle conditions such as Cerebral Palsy or Muscular Dystrophy. This is why prompt medical assessment by an individual's GP is essential in suspected cases of Scoliosis.

There is a form of Scoliosis that affects older people. We've all seen little old ladies or men with visibly curved spines. This is known as Degenerative Scoliosis and is thought to be caused by wear and tear of the spine over a lifetime in combination and bad posture.

Treatment options are more limited, due to the fact the spine has stopped growing and due to the higher risks associated with surgery in older people.

The main Degenerative Scoliosis is to prevent and minimise damage for as long as possible. This can be done by adopting a good posture and regular exercise - particularly that involves movement and flexibility of the spine.

Treatment for any pain caused by Degenerative Scoliosis is medication in the form of painkillers. Occasionally injections of steroids and local anaesthetics can help with nerve pain, but the effect of these is very short term (relief from the pain is only for 1-2 weeks).

In rare cases surgical options for Degenerative Scoliosis may be considered as a last resort (failure of all other treatment options). This relies on a number of factors, but generally the individual needs to be in a good state of health and that it is having a significant impact on the individual's quality of life.

Spinal Stenosis is a narrowing of the spinal canal which is where nerve tissue sits and spreads out from there. The spinal canal goes from the brainstem all the way down to the bottom of the spine. Nerves allow us to feel touch, heat and pain. When the spinal cord is narrowed such as in Spinal Stenosis nerves get compressed, causing pain, pins and needles or complete loss of sensation.

Spinal Stenosis can occur gradually or suddenly and can have a number of causes. Causes of gradual Spinal Stenosis include gradual narrowing due to age, being overweight, growth of tumours, Herniated (Slipped) Disk, fractures of vertebrae.

Sudden Spinal Stenosis can be caused by traumatic injury to the spine or Cauda Equina Syndrome. Immediate and emergency medical treatment should be sought for any sudden Spinal Stenosis.

Cauda Equina Syndrome is a rare condition characterised by numbness below the waist, loss of bladder control, some or complete loss of bowel control and loss of sensation to genitals. Cauda Equina Syndrome is a sudden compression of nerves. Cauda Equina Syndrome is a time sensitive condition. The longer it is left untreated the increased likelihood that the symptoms become permanent and irreversible. Treatment is emergency surgery by a team of Neurologists to relieve the pressure on the nerves.

Chapter 5 - The Muscular System

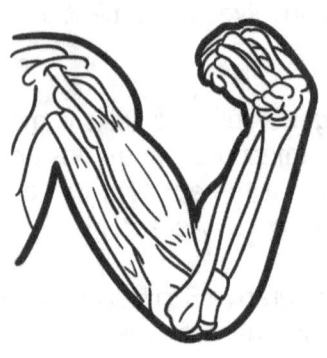

Bicep/Tricep Muscles.

Muscles enable movement. They enable two of my favourite things: eating and dancing. I learned during my childhood, that doing these two activities together, at the same time, isn't a good idea. It leads to vomiting.

More than 600 muscles make up the Muscular System. Motor Neurone Disease (MND) is an umbrella term to describe a number of conditions that affect functioning of muscles. Perhaps the most famous person with MND is the deceased Theoretical Physicist Dr Stephen Hawkins.

Although MND is a condition of the brain and nerves, I have chosen to place it in the Muscular System of this book because of the impact it has on this particular system. MND is caused by a group of neuron cells in the brain (called motor neurons), which are responsible for instructing muscles to move. These motor neurons gradually stop functioning.

It is not known why MND happens and there is no cure. It is a progressive disease that eventually leads to an individual losing complete muscle control. The amount of time this takes seems to vary from individual to individual. Sadly, people with MND have a shortened life expectancy and a significantly reduced quality of life.

Symptoms of MND include difficulty walking, weakness in hands, arms and legs, slurred speech, difficulties eating and swallowing and overtime weight loss.

Treatment for MND is a multidisciplinary team approach. It involves Consultant Neurologists (specialist Doctors), MND Specialist Nurses, Physiotherapists, Occupational Therapists, Speech & Language Therapists, Dieticians, Counsellors, Carers and Social Workers.

The aims of treatment are to minimise the impact MND has on the person's life and support carers/relatives.

Treatments include: medications, regular physio and occupational therapy, swallowing assessments, prescribed vitamin and mineral supplements, advice around diet and eating, speech and language therapy and counselling to help individuals deal with the mental and emotional impact of MND.

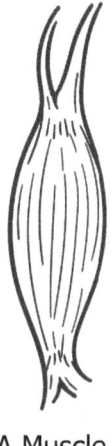

A Muscle.

Muscular Dystrophy (MD) is a number of genetic conditions that cause changes to the muscles, eventually rendering them unable to function. The type of MD usually determines its severity and the symptoms likely to be experienced.

But symptoms can include difficulty mobilising including walking like a drunk person, muscle pain and stiffness, delayed growth and in reaching developmental milestones, require support to complete activities of daily living, difficulties eating and drinking and possible learning disabilities.

There are no cures for MD conditions. Treatments include: medications (including steroids), physiotherapy, occupational therapy, dietician input, swallowing assessments, counselling or CBT (to support people with MD to deal with the mental and emotional aspects of having MD), support for carers/relatives, social work input and surgery.

Genetic testing and counselling is available for prospective parents who have MD in their family. The aim of these interventions are to minimise the risk of a baby being born with MD. But testing doesn't guarantee a baby will be born without MD and carries a small risk of miscarriage.

There is ongoing research into better treatments and possible cures for MD, looking at MD from a range of different angles.

Myasthenia Gravis is caused by a faulty immune system. White blood cells identify nerve and muscle cells, disrupting communication between them. Myasthenia Gravis can affect any part of the body, but most commonly affects the eyes, eyelids and muscles of the face (including those involved with chewing, swallowing and speaking).

Symptoms of Myasthenia Gravis include droopy eyelids, double vision, facial expression, problems with eating and drinking and weakness of the arms, legs and neck. Very occasionally Myasthenia Gravis can result in breathing difficulties, in these cases medical attention should be sought immediately.

There is no cure for Myasthenia Gravis. For some people with Myasthenia Gravis, symptoms are limited to the eyes, for others it gradually spreads throughout the body as time progresses.

Myasthenia Gravis has episodes where it flares-up. These episodes can be triggered by things like stress or tiredness. Treatments include identifying triggers and avoiding them, medications (including steroids, immune system suppressants and annual flu vaccinations) and sometimes surgery. It should be noted that non-reversible surgery isn't always successful at resolving symptoms and carries its own risks.

Myositis is a number of conditions which cause muscles to weaken over time. The exact cause of Myositis is not known. Some theorise that there might be a genetic link, as it tends to run in families.

Others theorise that some forms of Myositis are autoimmune conditions, meaning that white blood cells attack muscle and joint cells. Both are probably true, but are lacking in specific details.

The main symptoms of Myositis conditions are repeated falls resulting in bone fractures, struggling to pick up or use things using the hand's fine motor skills, painful muscles, swelling, fatigue and problems with swallowing and or breathing.

No cure exists for Myositis conditions. Myositis is treated with medications (including steroids, painkillers, anti-inflammatories & immunosuppressants), physiotherapy, speech and language input and occasionally immunoglobulin therapy. Immunoglobulin therapy involves using antibodies taken from blood donors to stabilise the immune system of the person with Myositis.

Parkinson's Disease is a condition where part of the brain becomes damaged over a long period of time. Although a neurological disease, the symptoms of it are present in the Muscular System. This is why I have listed it in this chapter. The symptoms of Parkinson's Disease include a tremor, muscle pain, stiffness, tension and reduced mobility and movement.

Scientists, Doctors and Researchers have all theorised and debated whether Parkinson's Disease is because of nature or nurture. Those in favour of nature argue that as it can run in families there must be genetics involved.

Those in favour of the nurture school of thought argue that environmental factors may increase someone's risk of developing Parkinson's Disease. They blame pesticides, herbicides and pollution.

No one argument is stronger than the other, as there is plenty of evidence against both of these theories.

Brain scans and developments in Neuroscience have identified what is going on in the brain with someone with Parkinson's Disease.

Parkinson's Disease is caused by the damage or death of neurons (brain cells) responsible for producing the chemical Dopamine. Dopamine is a messenger chemical, which helps control and coordinate movement. This causes a reduction of Dopamine in the brain and the presentation of the disease's symptoms.

An Dopamine Tangent:

In my book Mental Health Wisdom (2019), I wrote about

Dopamine:

Dopamine - The motivation chemical. It not only motivates you, but makes you feel good. It is made in the brain.

Dopamine motivates you to seek out things you need for your individual and species survival. Such as food, water and sex. It does this by operating a reward pathway. When your brain gets whatever the dopamine has motivated you to seek out, it stimulates the release of more dopamine across the lobes of the brain. This dopamine makes you feel really good. This rewards the behaviour and makes you more likely to repeat it.

Never underestimate just how good dopamine can make you feel.

Dopamine and its reward pathway are thought to be the physiological cause of addictions to substances, ultimately destructive behaviours (such as gambling or eating too much) and even the high you get following a good session of exercise at the gym.

It was a surprise to learn about Dopamine's role in Parkinson's Disease. It just goes to show that humans have a very limited understanding of how the arguably most important organ in the body, the brain, functions.

It's no surprise, given the Dopamine Tangent above that symptoms of Parkinson's Disease can also include anxiety and depression.

There is no cure for Parkinson's Disease and it gets worse as time progresses. Treatments include medications (medications to increase dopamine levels in the brain, antidepressants and other medications to help manage symptoms), physiotherapy, occupational therapy, dietician input, speech & language therapy and surgery.

Osteoarthritis is a condition in which joints become stiff causing reduced mobility and severe pain in areas of the body affected. Joints don't actually sit under the muscular system, but Osteoarthritis has been included in this chapter because of the symptoms that people with Osteoarthritis experience.

Symptoms of Osteoarthritis include decreased ability to move, severe pain, sometimes swelling to affected parts of the body and sometimes bony growths. The cause of Osteoarthritis isn't known or fully understood.

But there are risk factors that seem to increase the risk of developing Osteoarthritis. These risk factors include:
* A previous joint injury.
* other conditions that damage joints.
* A family history of Osteoarthritis, suggesting a genetic link in some cases.
* Obesity, as the additional weight puts more strain on the joints.
* Being female, Osteoarthritis is more prevalent in females than in males.
* Being older in age, possibly due to wear and tear.

Preventing Osteoarthritis involves reducing the risk factors above. There is no cure for Osteoarthritis. However Osteoarthritis doesn't always get worse as time progresses and can sometimes improve over time.

Treatments for Osteoarthritis involve painkillers, physiotherapy and very occasionally surgery to repair or replace damaged joints.

A Hernia is when a part of the body pushes through a weakness in the muscular system. There are a number of different types of hernias depending where on the body they appear. A hernia becomes a medical emergency if the following symptoms are being experienced: sudden severe pain, nausea/vomiting, the hernia becomes tender/painful to touch and difficulty opening bowels. In these cases urgent surgery is required to prevent bowel obstructions or the blood supply being cut off to the affected part of the body.

Chapter 6 - The Lymphatic & Immune Systems

The immune system is made up of the lymphatic system (bone marrow, lymph nodes, thymus, spleen and lymphatic vessels). It's a complex system and a lot can go wrong with it. All the diseases and conditions in this chapter are caused by malfunctions of the lymphatic and immune systems.

Harmful Organisms
There are three types of harmful organisms that are worth knowing about that can invade and infect the human body:

1. Bacteria - These are organisms that can be killed by both the immune system and antibiotic medications.

2. Viruses - These are organisms that can be killed by the immune system, but don't respond to antibiotic medications. In life threatening situations, antiviral medications can be given that stop or slow down the multiplication of viruses. This gives the body's immune system a fighting chance.

3. Fungi - These are caused by yeast or mould. Many people think that these sorts of infections can only affect skin or nails. But they can grow in any moist areas of the body including mouth, throat, lungs, urinary tract, vagina, penis and genital areas of both males and females.

A Bacteria Cell.

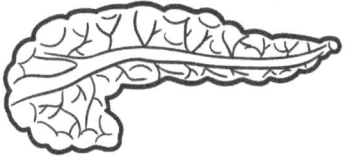

The Pancreas.

There are three types of Diabetes, Type 1, Type 2 and Gestational (develops during Pregnancy). Before I explain the three types of diabetes, it is important to understand the role of insulin in the body. Insulin is a hormone made in the Pancreas that is required by every cell in the human body to function. Insulin allows glucose from dietary intake to enter cells to be used as energy.

In Type 1 Diabetes, white blood cells (these fight foreign organisms in the body such as bacteria and viruses) mistake insulin producing cells in the pancreas as being foreign and attack them. These vital insulin producing cells get destroyed and no longer function.

This leads to a high blood sugar (medical term: Hyperglycemia). Symptoms of a high blood sugar include extreme and unquenchable thirst, dry mouth, increased urination frequency and amount, fatigue and the feeling of always being tired (no matter how much the person sleeps), repeated thrush (in both males and females), occasionally blurred vision, weight loss and sweet smelling breath.

High blood sugar can potentially lead to a condition called Diabetic Ketoacidosis (DKA). DKA is caused by a lack of insulin in the body. When the body doesn't have enough insulin, the liver converts fat cells into energy for cells throughout the body. A byproduct of this process is the release of harmful ketones into the bloodstream.

DKA can be life threatening and medical attention should be sought as soon as possible, as DKA gets worse without treatment as time passes. DKA isn't a condition in itself, more a potential consequence of diabetes. It is treated with intravenous insulin and fluids to replace those lost and prevent dehydration.

Diabetes is diagnosed through a finger prick blood test with near instant results and a regular blood test to confirm. There is no cure for Type 1 Diabetes, although several are being worked on across the world. A person can become Type 1 Diabetic at any age, although it is more commonly diagnosed in childhood.

Treatments for Type 1 Diabetes are constantly evolving, but all have two main components: monitoring blood sugars and administration of insulin subcutaneously (giving insulin via a needle under the skin or via an insulin pump). Occasionally other medications aimed at lowering blood sugars may also be prescribed.

Managing blood sugars in Type 1 Diabetes is key to preventing complications that the long term chronic disease can bring such as blindness, high blood pressure, high cholesterol, loss of sensation or pain in peripheral nerves, loss of toes/feet/legs due to circulation problems and kidney problems.

The problem with Type 1 Diabetes comes with the number of influences on blood sugar levels including: the amount of carbohydrates eaten, the amount of insulin administered, mental health illnesses, stress, the weather, exercise, other illnesses or infections, surgery, hormonal changes. Practically anything really can influence the blood sugars of an individual with Type 1 diabetes.

This can make someone living with Type 1 Diabetes feel like their diabetes is a two year old child, unpredictable and likely to play up when you least want it to.

Low blood sugars (medical term: Hypoglycemia) can occur in people with Type 1 Diabetes occurring due to too much insulin being present in the body. Symptoms of a low blood sugar include shaking, sweats, hunger, feeling weak/tired, heart palpitations, collapse (late symptom) and seizures (late symptom). Some people with Type 1 Diabetes lose their awareness of low blood sugar symptoms as time passes.

Low blood sugars are easily treated by the individual with Type 1 Diabetes by them eating some fast acting sugars, followed by some food with slower acting carbohydrates.

Type 2 Diabetes is not related to the immune system, but it made sense to include it here. Type 2 Diabetes is thought to be caused by either old age or obesity.

In the case of old age, it is theorised that the insulin producing cells in the pancreas are worn out and no longer produce enough insulin for all the cells in the body. With obesity, there are just too many cells for the insulin producing cells to produce insulin for.

Type 2 Diabetes is usually identified by a routine blood test. But some people are identified by symptoms of a high blood sugar (see above).

With Type 2 Diabetes the initial treatment is usually changes to diet and lifestyle (exercising regularly and losing weight). Sometimes these changes on their own are enough to manage Type 2 Diabetes and in some cases reverse it.

If the changes to diet and lifestyle are ineffective at managing Type 2 Diabetes, medications are prescribed to reduce the blood sugar. It can take time to find the right medication(s) and dosage. These medications are usually effective in managing blood sugars in people with Type 2 Diabetes. On rare occasions where these medications are not effective, the final option is insulin, injected subcutaneously.

Gestational Diabetes develops during pregnancy. It can develop at any point during the pregnancy and any pregnant woman can develop it. It is caused because the body can't produce enough insulin to meet the extra needed during pregnancy. Most women with Gestational Diabetes initially have no symptoms, however some women do develop symptoms associated with a high blood sugar (see symptoms above).

In the UK, all women who have one or more of the following risk factors are screened for Gestational Diabetes:
- A woman that has had Gestational Diabetes in a previous pregnancy.
- A woman who has previously given birth to a baby who weighed 4.5KGS or more at birth.
- A woman who has a parent or sibling with any type of diabetes.
- A woman that has a Body Mass Index (BMI) above 30.
- A woman who has had any weight loss surgery, including a gastric bypass.
- A woman that is over 40 years old at time of pregnancy.
- Any woman of the following ethnicities (even if they were born in the UK): South Asian, Black, African-Caribbean or Middle Eastern origin.

Screening for Gestational Diabetes is really easy and is called an Oral Glucose Tolerance Test. It is really important that Gestational Diabetes is identified and treated. Gestational Diabetes can have an impact on the pregnancy and the unborn baby, particularly if it isn't identified and treated.

Treating Gestational Diabetes lowers the risk of a baby being born bigger than normal - causing complications during labour, premature birth, too much fluid in the womb (medical term: polyhydramnios), high blood pressure during pregnancy (medical term: pre-eclampsia) and a baby being born with low blood sugar and being yellow (medical term: jaundice) at birth both requiring medical treatment. On very rare occasions untreated Gestational Diabetes and associated complications can lead to a stillbirth.

Treatment for Gestational Diabetes is monitoring of blood sugar levels, changes to diet and gentle exercise. If these are ineffective then medications to bring down the high blood sugar levels may be prescribed. Sometimes it is necessary to have insulin prescribed subcutaneously to manage blood sugar levels.

People with Type 2 Diabetes and Gestational Diabetes can have low blood sugars caused by too much insulin in the body. The symptoms of low blood sugar and treatment are the same in all types of Diabetes (see above for more details of low blood sugars).

There is good news with Gestational Diabetes. Unlike Type 1 and Type 2 Diabetes that are conditions that people generally have for life, Gestational Diabetes usually resolves after the birth of the baby. The monitoring of blood sugars and treatments are no longer required.

For more details about the pancreas see p88-89.

Lupus is a complex autoimmune condition where white blood cells attack various parts of the body. The cause of Lupus is currently unknown. Some researchers suggest that it could be genetic, others that it is a mix of genetics and environmental factors. Lupus can occur at any age and be categorised by its severity.

Mild Lupus brings symptoms of fatigue, skin problems and stiff, achy or painful joints. Moderate Lupus causes inflammation to the skin and some organs such as the heart, lungs and kidneys. Severe Lupus can be life threatening by causing swelling and damage to the brain, heart, lungs and kidneys.

Lupus usually occurs in episodes and then goes into remission. It is not fully known what triggers these episodes in Lupus. Current treatment for Lupus is medications to manage symptoms, for example anti-inflammatory medications for swelling, painkillers for pain and often steroids. Sometimes immunosuppressant medications are used to reduce the activity of the immune system.

Specialist input from Consultants in Neurology (brain), Cardiac (heart), Respiratory (lungs) and Endocrine (kidneys) may be required to assess, treat and manage the damage caused by Lupus.

Lupus is a lifelong condition and can have a significant impact on an individual's physical and mental health.

Multiple Sclerosis (MS) is a condition where the white blood cells attack the brain and spinal cord. This assault on the nervous system results in the following symptoms:

- ❖ Fatigue, no matter how well rested an individual is.
- ❖ Muscle stiffness or pain - this is due to nerve damage and can be experienced anywhere in the body.
- ❖ Eye problems such as blurred vision, temporary loss of sight and painful eyes (worse on movement).
- ❖ Problems in the frontal lobe of the brain - the part of the brain associated with planning, risk assessment and logic. This may also affect the ability to remember new things and learn new information.
- ❖ Reduced mobility and sometimes a reduced ability to undertake tasks involving hand-eye coordination.
- ❖ Reduced ability to control bladder and bowels, leading to incidents of incontinence.
- ❖ Mental illness - depression and anxiety.
- ❖ Speech and swallowing problems.
- ❖ Loss of interest in sex and other difficulties in this area.

People with MS either have symptomatic episodes (known as 'Relapsing Remitting MS') or have constant symptoms (known as 'Primary Progressive MS').

People with MS who have symptomatic episodes have periods of remission (being symptom free). In these cases another symptomatic episode could happen at any time, without any warning.

People with constant MS symptoms have no periods of remission, although there are periods when the symptoms appear to somewhat stabilise. In these cases, the symptoms gradually get worse as the years pass.

Both types of MS significantly affect people's quality of life and mental health.

MS is theorised to be genetic as it often runs in families and it is also theorised to be triggered by certain external factors. There is some evidence to support this theory but it is far from being conclusive.

There is no cure for MS. Treatments depend on symptoms but always include a multidisciplinary team (MDT) approach. Medications including steroids are used to manage symptoms, as are physiotherapy, occupational therapy, specialist pain management nurses, incontinence nurses, mental health professionals, social work input and on some occasions input from a sex therapist.

Rheumatoid Arthritis is a condition where those pesky white blood cells of the immune system get it wrong and attack cells near joints. Joints are at the end of bones and enable movement of the skeletal system. In Rheumatoid Arthritis the attacked joints become swollen, painful, stiff, difficult to move and over time become damaged.

The cause of Rheumatoid Arthritis is unknown and there isn't a cure. The key with Rheumatoid Arthritis is early diagnosis. This enables treatments to reduce the symptoms and prevent the damage to joints for as long as possible. Treatments include medications (including steroids and painkillers), physiotherapy, occupational therapy, podiatry and as the disease progresses surgery.

Sjögren Syndrome is a condition where the white blood cells attack cells that produce bodily fluids. The white blood cells damage the cells resulting in them no longer being able to function. This causes dry eyes, mouth, dry skin, muscle/joint pain, vaginal dryness in females, thrush in both genders and fatigue. Sjögren Syndrome can vary in severity from mild to severe.

Some people with Sjögren Syndrome have other autoimmune conditions (see above). Sjögren Syndrome can sometimes affect other parts of the body such as nerves. The exact cause of Sjögren Syndrome is unknown and treatments are symptom-based. For example, if an individual has dry eyes, eye drops can be used, taking regular breaks from screens and attending regular Optician appointments.

In Pernicious Anaemia white blood cells attack cells in the stomach that produce a protein called intrinsic factor. Intrinsic factor is required to allow the absorption of iron (Vitamin B12) into the body. This leads to low iron levels (medical term: Anaemia) in the body.

It is worth noting that Pernicious Anaemia is not the only cause of low iron levels. Anaemia can also be caused by poor diet, some conditions affecting the stomach or intestines, conditions that increase urination (the frequency of peeing), some medications or the increased demand for iron during pregnancy.

The exact cause of Pernicious Anaemia is unknown and there isn't a cure. Symptoms of Pernicious Anaemia include fatigue, being short of breath, headaches, loss of appetite, palpitations, problems with eyesight and sometimes cognitive impairment.

Treatment for Pernicious Anaemia involves replacing the Vitamin B12 that the body is not absorbing through regular injections of Vitamin B12.

The Spleen is a small cylindrical shaped organ that sits on the left side of the Stomach, protected by the rib cage in humans. The Spleen has several main functions:

❖ White blood cells - It creates a specific type of white cells called Lymphocytes to combat harmful bacterial and viral cells.

❖ Antibodies - It creates antibodies based on past bacterial and viral infections. An antibody is a blood protein that enables white blood cells to identify and therefore counteract harmful cells.

❖ It acts as a filter, removing potentially harmful cells from the blood.

❖ Red blood cells - It creates red blood cells and removes damaged or old red blood cells from circulation in the bloodstream.

❖ Platelets - It stores platelets and releases them into the bloodstream as required.

❖ Stabilises Levels - It stabilises levels of red and white blood cells and platelets in the bloodstream. This includes increasing or decreasing levels depending on what is required in the body. So if for example an individual has an infection, the Spleen will respond by increasing the number of white blood cells in the body to respond.

These functions make the Spleen pretty important in maintaining a good immune response. But interestingly someone can survive and live without a Spleen. In these cases the Liver takes on some of the functions of the Spleen.

The Spleen doesn't get enough credit as an organ in the human body. Some people don't even realise that it exists, let alone that it works tirelessly like a workhorse. It is generally pretty reliable, but there are a few things that can go wrong with it.

On rare occasions a baby can be born without a Spleen (medical term: Asplenia). As previously written people can live without a Spleen. There isn't an explanation or theory as to why a baby might be born without a Spleen.

The main risk with not having a Spleen (at any age) or having a Spleen that doesn't function as it should is a serious and potentially life threatening infection. Prompt medical treatment in these cases saves lives.

Thinking about the functions of the Spleen (above), one that isn't working properly (also known as a damaged Spleen, medical term: Hyposplenism) can lead to:

❖ A reduced number of red blood cells (medical term: Anaemia). This can lead to symptoms that include: fatigue, shortness of breath and heart palpitations.

❖ A reduced number of white blood cells. This can lead to recurrent infections or increased risk of serious infections.

❖ Low numbers of platelets. This leads to slower blood clotting in the event of a bleed. This is particularly important during surgical procedures (whether emergency or planned) and in the event of an accident. Symptoms of low platelets can include a higher risk of bruising.

Sometimes people can experience a painful Spleen. This can be a symptom of a damaged, enlarged or ruptured Spleen.

An enlarged Spleen is usually caused by injury or infection. It can sometimes be a symptom of another underlying condition.

Sometimes there are no symptoms of an enlarged Spleen. Other times there are. Symptoms can include feeling full easily when eating (due to the Spleen putting pressure on the Stomach), pain or discomfort in the area where the Spleen is located, fatigue with a low red blood cell count, recurring infections and bruising easily.

Treatment for an enlarged Spleen is to treat the underlying cause of it. So if a bacterial infection is the cause, for example, intravenous antibiotics should be administered. An enlarged Spleen is usually monitored and resolves once the underlying cause is treated.

A ruptured spleen is where the spleen bursts and is no longer able to function normally. A ruptured spleen is caused by traumatic injury usually through car accidents or sports injuries. A ruptured spleen usually causes pain, but due to the accident or injury an individual is unable to distinguish the cause of the pain.

A ruptured spleen causes internal bleeding and can be fatal if not immediately treated. Sometimes the rupture can be large causing a large amount of blood loss internally very quickly. Sometimes it can be a smaller rupture causing more gradual blood loss.

Symptoms of significant blood loss include:
❖ An increased pulse (this is considered to be a heart rate of more than 100 beats per minute, medical term: Tachycardia).

❖ A falling blood pressure (in the case of a large rupture this will happen very quickly, medical term: Hypotension).

❖ Dizziness.

❖ Confusion.

❖ Blurred vision.

❖ Anxiety or agitation.

❖ In some cases Nausea.

If the cardiovascular system loses enough blood, it will go into Cardiogenic Shock resulting in a cardiac arrest.

The treatments for a ruptured Spleen include blood transfusions, intravenous fluids and rapid surgery.

A damaged, enlarged or ruptured spleen sometimes needs to be surgically removed, in part or in whole (medical term: Splenectomy).

Types of White Blood Cells

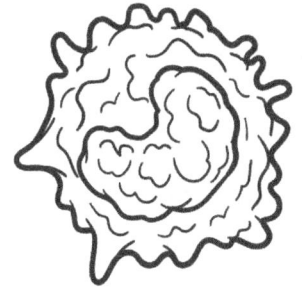

A Monocyte

There are different types of White Blood Cells and it can be useful to know the different types and how they work:

❖ Monocytes - These float around the body identifying and destroying harmful cells and cells that have been infected by these harmful cells.

❖ Lymphocytes - These create antibodies so that other white blood cells can identify foreign cells that the immune system has past experience with.

❖ Neutrophils - These cells are the first line of defence in your immune system and literally consume harmful cells.

❖ Basophils - These cells sound the alarm when they detect harmful cells, alerting other white blood cells to the presence of harmful cells. Imagine them waving and shouting: OVER HERE! AN INTRUDER!

❖ Eosinophils - These cells specialise in dealing with parasites and cancer cells. They also assist in the immune system's responses to allergies.

Anaphylactic Shock
Anaphylactic shock is caused by a severe overreaction to an external stimuli (such a bee/wasp sting or ingestion of peanuts) from the immune system. The immune system suddenly floods the cardiovascular system with chemicals that cause the body to go into shock. In a matter of minutes someone can go from being fine to being in Anaphylactic shock.

The best treatment for Anaphylactic shock is administration of adrenaline via an Epipen. Epipens really do save lives.

If I had my way, I'd have them in every restaurant and public space possible, a bit like the way Defibrillators are becoming commonplace in public spaces.

Septic Shock
Septic shock is caused by an infection in the body.

Joke:
Doctor: "You're very unwell."
Patient: "Can I get a second opinion?"
Doctor: "Okay, you're very ugly as well."

Chapter 7 - The Respiratory System

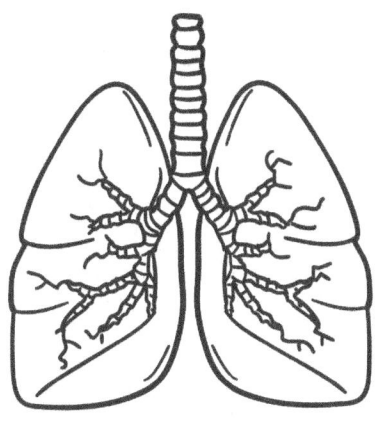

The Lungs.

The Respiratory System is made up of the lungs and the pharynx. Most people are familiar with the lungs and their functions of inhaling oxygen and exhaling carbon dioxide.

But people are less familiar with the pharynx. The pharynx is part of the throat behind the mouth and nasal cavity. It has a dual function. It allows air down through the Larynx (known also as the voice box) and into a tube called the Trachea, which then flows Bronchi (smaller tubes) down through the Bronchioles (even smaller tubes) and into the Alveoli where the gases of oxygen and carbon dioxide are exchanged.

The pharynx's other function is to allow chewed food, fluids and oral medications taken in the mouth to pass through it into the oesophagus (the tube down to the stomach). For more information see chapter 10 - The Gastrointestinal System on p89-101.

Although the nose is placed in The Sensory Organs System chapter of this book, it also has functions in The Respiratory System. The nose helps to provide air inhaled with humidity, warmth and filters it.

The Respiratory System like every other system in the body can go wrong.

Asthma is a relatively common condition of the lungs. In asthma, the airways are affected by swelling and the development of mucus. The exact cause of asthma is unknown and there isn't a cure for Asthma, only treatments.

Symptoms of an asthma attack are shortness of breath, tightness of the chest, coughing, fast heart rate, blueness of the lips/fingers and sometimes confusion. Treatments include medications (including steroids) usually delivered directly to the affected airways by inhaler or nebuliser. In some cases surgery may be recommended.

Asthma attacks are sometimes triggered by certain things like a smoky environment, infections, certain medications, emotions, the weather, exercise, allergies to just name a few. Asthma attacks can develop suddenly over a short space of time or more slowly and gradually over days. Asthma attacks can be life threatening and early treatment can save lives.

Cystic Fibrosis (CF) is a genetic condition which is caused by a faulty gene inherited from an individual's biological parents. There isn't a cure for CF, however it can be identified early through genetic testing. CF results in a buildup of mucus in the lungs and organs involved in the digestion of food. CF is a progressive disease, meaning that it gets worse as time progresses.

Symptoms of CF include failure to thrive (in babies and young children), repeated chest infections, shortness of breath, weight loss, signs of malnutrition, jaundice and problems with bowel movements (constipation or loose bowel movements).

Care for people with CF is through a multidisciplinary team (MDT) approach. Treatments include daily physiotherapy to try to cough up and clear the lungs of mucus, medications (including antibiotics and steroids), dietitian input, Respiratory Consultant & Specialist Nurse reviews and sometimes Social Work input.

At some point people with CF may be offered a lung transplant, subject to the deteriorating state of their lungs and availability of lungs for transplant. There are significant risks associated with lung transplant surgery, however if successful, can greatly improve an individual's quality of life and ability to breathe.

Pulmonary Embolism (PE) is a medical term for a blood clot forming in one of the blood vessels in the lungs. There is no one single cause of a PE, but instead risk factors that increase the likelihood of having a PE.

These factors can include a person who has cancer/is undergoing cancer treatment, some cardiovascular conditions (such as heart failure, high blood pressure and high cholesterol) and certain medications (the increased risks of PE should be discussed with an individual before they are commenced on these medications).

Although this is an issue in the cardiovascular system, I have chosen to include it here due to the system affected. The symptoms of a PE include chest pain, difficulty breathing and in some (but not all cases) coughing up fresh blood. Symptoms of a PE may come on suddenly or gradually over days, getting worse as time progresses.

A PE is treated with anticoagulant medications. The aim of treatment is to safely break down the blood clot, stopping the blood flow from being impeded. The treatment also can prevent future clots from developing in the cardiovascular system.

Sleep Apnea is when breathing stops during sleep. In babies and young children sleep apnea is thought to be caused by an immaturity of the brain stem. Essentially the brain forgets to send messages to the lungs to tell them to breathe during sleep. Although this can be very scary for parents/carers, stimulation to the babies' body through touch triggers the brain to resume breathing.

Sleep Apnea monitors can be bought for babies and young children. These are also used in medical settings such as Children's Wards and Special Care Baby Units (as premature babies are at increased risk of Sleep Apnea). The great news is that as babies or young children continue to grow and get older, this immaturity in the brain step resolves itself without the need for ongoing treatment or care.

The cause of Sleep Apnea in adults is not fully understood. But there are lifestyle risk factors that increase risk of an individual developing Sleep Apnea including being overweight, alcohol use and smoking.

The symptoms of Sleep Apnea include feeling tired, waking up a lot during the night - usually for unexplained reasons, finding it difficult to concentrate, regular headaches and sometimes mood swings. If someone has a partner, it is usually their partner that will notice that they snore loudly, stop breathing, making gasping or choking noises during the night.

Treatments start with lifestyle changes. If these are ineffective then using a CPAP (Continuous Positive Airway Pressure) Machine during sleep may be required. Very occasionally surgery may be required.

Sleep Apnea can be debilitating for an individual to live with. It can cause relationship issues, increase the risk of physical and mental diseases and puts them at a higher risk of accidents due to extreme tiredness.

Tuberculosis (TB) is a serious bacterial infection of the lungs. Some people who are at high risk of TB are given a vaccine to prevent them from getting it. TB can be symptomatic (also known as Active TB) or have no symptoms (also known as Latent TB).

Children and young people with TB tend to have difficulties growing and developing. TB symptoms in adults tend to include extreme exhaustion, a cough lasting more than two weeks (any cough lasting more than two weeks should always be checked out by a medical professional), a high temperature, loss of appetite with or without weight loss and feeling generally unwell.

Like any infection, TB can start in an individual's lungs and then spread to other parts of the body. If TB spreads individuals may experience other symptoms, related to where TB has spread. For example, if it has spread to a joint, the joint may swell and become painful.

TB is treated with long term antibiotics (for at least 6 months, but usually more) and medications to treat and ease symptoms (including steroids).

Today, TB is uncommon in the UK due to vaccinations, improved identification, improved treatment and improved awareness around infection prevention measures, such as hand washing. However, TB is very prevalent in certain parts of the world and should be considered if anyone has been on holiday abroad/travelled abroad recently or is from another country.

A Pneumothorax is when air leaks out of the lungs into the chest cavity and chest wall. It is sometimes known as collapsed lung because the leaking air causes pressure to build up so that the lung can't expand as it normally would on inhalation. There are a number of potential causes of Pneumothorax including:

❖ A blister on the surface of the lung has burst, creating a hole in the lung that allows the air to leak. With this cause, the blister was present on the lung from birth. There is often no reason why the blister bursts when it does.

❖ Certain conditions such as Chronic Obstructive Pulmonary Disease (COPD) can increase the risk of Pneumothorax occurring.

❖ Injury or trauma to the chest. The rib cage is there to protect the lungs and heart, but the rib cage is not a perfect system. If significant pressure is put on the rib cage, it can be crushed and damage the lungs. The sort of injuries where you would need to consider Pneumothorax include road traffic accidents, falls (particularly falls from a height), accidents resulting from some outdoor activities (such as rock climbing & rafting) and significant assaults/attacks - particularly with weapons.

❖ Injury to lungs from medical care or treatment, such as taking biopsies from the lungs or draining fluid from the lungs.

The symptoms of a Pneumothorax are shortness of breath, chest pain (sometimes worse on breathing or coughing), fatigue, elevated respiratory rate and sometimes a dry cough.

Treatment for a Pneumothorax depends on how big the hole is in the lung and how much air has leaked out into the chest cavity and chest wall.

If the hole is small with the air having a minimal impact on the operation of the lung (particularly its ability to expand) an individual will usually be given medications to relieve pain and be invited to a follow-up clinic to ensure that the hole has healed and the lung is functioning normally.

If the leaked air is causing significant pressure on the lung and is affecting its ability to function an aspiration may be required to remove the air. An aspiration involves putting a needle through the chest into the space between the chest wall and lung, in order to remove the air. This is generally done under local anaesthetic.

In the case of a severe Pneumothorax, sometimes a chest drain is needed. A chest drain is a tube inserted into the chest, which will allow the air to leave the chest cavity.

The hole in the lung eventually heals on its own, but this does take time.

COPD is an umbrella term to describe a number of conditions that affect the function of the Respiratory System. In COPD conditions damage occurs to the airways leading to permanent inflammation and narrowing. This damage usually occurs over years and people don't realise they have COPD until they begin to develop symptoms.

In the medical and nursing professions people tend to think of COPD as only having one cause: smoking. It's true that smoking is a known cause of COPD and is usually the cause in most cases of COPD. But people can get COPD from long term exposure to some chemicals (in certain work environments) and some rare genetic conditions.

Nicotine Dependency
This book is about the ways that the body can go wrong. I have deliberately excluded things that humans do to their own bodies, to prevent this book from becoming a health encyclopaedia.

However I do want to remind my health professional colleagues of our requirement to have a non-judgemental approach, of our responsibility towards public health work (every contact is an opportunity to improve the health of the individual) and that Nicotine is a severely addictive drug.

I have worked in dependency services for well over a decade. By far the hardest drug to give up and stay abstinent from is Nicotine.

The best way to treat Nicotine Dependency currently is with a combination of medications (whether this be Nicotine Replacement Therapy, e-cigs/vapes or some of the newer medications that work in the brain) and Specialist Support.

I should add here that I am not advocating a particular approach, the approach should depend on the needs and wishes of the individual and be inline with local treatment policies.

COPD can have no symptoms for years, but this doesn't mean the damage is not being done to the Respiratory System. When COPD symptoms do appear they can be gradual or sudden. Symptoms include becoming short of breath - particularly when undertaking physically active tasks such as walking, recurrent chest infections, a cough that doesn't go away and sometimes a wheeze when breathing.

There is no cure for COPD and it progressive, meaning that it gets worse with time. Giving up smoking is the first recommendation to prevent/slow further damage. Other than that, the treatment is to manage symptoms and includes medications (including inhalers, steroids, oxygen, nebulisers & in the case of bacterial infections antibiotics).

Pneumonia is a particular nasty airborne bacteria or virus that can be life threatening for vulnerable people (the young, the elderly, those with a weak immune system and those with other chronic diseases). There is no cure for Pneumonia but there is a vaccination that protects against catching Pneumonia that is recommended for vulnerable people.

Symptoms of Pneumonia include elevated respiratory rate, shortness of breath, high temperature, chest pain, aches and pains, loss of appetite and exhaustion - leading to difficulties with the tasks of daily living and confusion (particularly as people get older).

Treatments for Pneumonia include antibiotics, steroids, intravenous fluids, anti inflammatory medications and paracetamol (to reduce a high temperature and manage any pain). Occasionally, antiviral medications may be used if viral Pneumonia is suspected and is life threatening. The infection usually resolves within a couple of weeks after treatment, however a full recovery from Pneumonia can take up to six months.

Pulmonary Edema is a build up of fluid in the lungs, which affects their ability to function. There are several causes of Pulmonary Edema, the most common cause is heart problems. Other causes of Pulmonary Edema include traumatic injury to the lungs, Pneumonia, exposure to certain toxins, some medications and travelling to or exercising at high altitude.

The development of a sudden Pulmonary Edema is life threatening and immediate medical treatment should be sought. Symptoms of Pulmonary Edema include shortness of breath - particularly when active, waking in the night feeling breathless and an increased difficulty in breathing if lay flat. Sometimes someone with Pulmonary Edema may also cough up fresh blood.

Pulmonary Edema is treated with oxygen, medications to remove the fluids from the lungs and sometimes medicines to help the heart function better.

Joke: Why did the lungs break up with the heart?
They just couldn't breathe anymore.

Chapter 8 - The Cardiovascular System

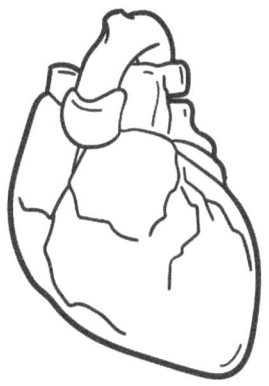

The Heart.

The Cardiovascular system is made up of the heart, blood vessels (including veins and arteries) and blood.

It is useful to start by understanding the makeup of the blood. The average adult has around 10 pints of blood that circulate around the human body.

Blood is made up of the following components:

❖ Plasma - Is the liquid part of the blood and enables travel around the body. It consists of a mixture of nutrients, waste products, sugar, fats, proteins, electrolytes and hormones. It also consists of red & white blood cells and platelets.

❖ Red Blood Cells - Carry oxygen to every cell in the human body and carry carbon dioxide back to the lungs for exhalation.

❖ White Blood Cells - Make up the immune system, see chapter 6 - The Lymphatic & Immune Systems p47-59 for further details.

❖ Platelets - Are responsible for clotting any holes or breaks in the blood vessels and essentially prevent an individual from losing all their blood in the event of a cut, graze or other trauma to the cardiovascular system (including medical interventions such as taking blood for testing).

Alcohol & Platelets
Although this book doesn't go into detail on failures of the human body caused by actions of humans, there is something worth noting about alcohol and platelets.

Alcohol is toxic to the bone marrow where platelets are made. Therefore people that drink heavily have a reduced number of platelets. This means that any break in the blood vessels will take longer to stop bleeding.

It takes 7-10 days following cessation of alcohol use to return to normal levels.

There is always blood loss during surgery (whether planned or emergency surgery). It is therefore important if having planned surgery to abstain from alcohol for 7-10 days prior to the date of surgery.

The cardiovascular system is complex and there's lots that can malfunction.

Electrolytes are minerals found in the bloodstream that enable the body to function normally. Whilst Electrolyte imbalances are not a condition in themselves, but usually a symptom of another condition, it is well worth being aware of Electrolytes.

Electrolyte imbalances can have serious consequences if not identified and treated, these consequences can include a irregular heartbeat (medical term: Arrhythmia), fast heart rate, fatigue, nausea and vomiting, headaches, seizures (potentially leading to death), abnormal bowel movements and muscle weakness/cramps/pain.

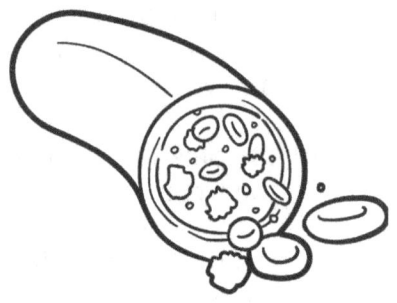

A blood vessel, sliced open showing the makeup of the blood.

Electrolytes in the blood include:
- ❖ Calcium
- ❖ Chloride
- ❖ Magnesium
- ❖ Phosphate

❖ Potassium
❖ Sodium

Treatments for Electrolyte imbalances involve treating any which are higher or lower than the normal range. High Electrolytes are treated by intravenous fluids and medications to reduce the high Electrolytes. Low Electrolytes are treated by giving the Electrolytes. It is important that the underlying cause of the Electrolyte imbalances are identified and treated.

Joke: The Doctor says: "Sorry, but your body has run out of magnesium."
Patient says: "0Mg."

As a good friend and former Nurse on a Coronary Care Unit once explained to me: There are two types of problems you get with the heart:
1. Problems with the pump (the muscle of the heart).
2. Problems with the electrics (the messages the brain sends to the heart to tell it to beat).

This is always useful to bear in mind when considering ways the heart and cardiovascular system can go wrong.

Cardiomyopathy is an umbrella term for diseases that affect the muscle of the heart. In Cardiomyopathy, the walls of the heart's chambers become stretched, thickened or stiff. This affects the heart's ability to effectively pump blood around the body. There are different types of Cardiomyopathy including:
❖ Dilated Cardiomyopathy - The walls of the heart become stretched and lead to the heart being ineffective at pumping blood around the body. It can affect both children and adults. With this type of Cardiomyopathy there is an increased risk of blood clots, arrhythmia (irregular heart beat) and it can progress on to heart failure.

❖ Hypertrophic Cardiomyopathy - The heart enlarges and its tissues thicken. The heart is less effective at pumping blood around the body. This type of Cardiomyopathy some people have no symptoms of and there is no impact on the activities of daily living. However it is not without risks. The risks with this type of Cardiomyopathy are extensive and include a leaky heart valve, irregular heart rhythms and can cause sudden and unexpected death in children and athletes.

❖ Restrictive Cardiomyopathy - This form of cardiomyopathy is rare and is where the walls of the heart become permanently stiff meaning that the chambers can't fill fully with blood. This leads to the heart being ineffective in pumping blood around the body. It can occur at any age. The cause is sometimes unknown, other times can be genetically inherited.

❖ Arrhythmogenic Cardiomyopathy (ACM) - Is a genetic condition caused by a protein that causes the heart structure to become stretched. ACM can also cause cell death in the cells and tissues that make up the muscles of the heart. This malfunction of the heart causes an irregular heart beat.

❖ Takotsubo Cardiomyopathy (also known as Broken Heart Syndrome) - A sudden burst of emotional tension or stress triggers this type of cardiomyopathy. So yes, medically I can tell you officially - you can physically have a broken heart. The good news with this type of cardiomyopathy is that it is temporary and heals itself over time.

There are no cures for any type of cardiomyopathy. Treatments include lifestyle changes, medications and sometimes surgery.

Angina is a condition caused by a reduced supply of blood to the heart. The main symptom of Angina is severe chest pain, to an individual it can often feel like having a heart attack and that they are going to die. With Angina, the pain usually resolves after several minutes of an individual resting.

Angina is often characterised as being stable or unstable. Stable angina has identifiable triggers such as stress or exercise. With unstable angina it can come on at random times and the pain continues for longer than in stable angina.

There is no cure for angina but medications can be used to treat it. Firstline treatment is x2 Glyceryl Trinitrate (GTN) Sprays, wait a few minutes, if no improvement, a further x2 GTN Sprays, if no improvement after a few minutes of the second GTN Sprays an ambulance should be called for immediate medical treatment.

Very occasionally surgery for angina may be required to improve the blood supply to the heart.

Endocarditis is an infection of the inner lining of the heart. It is caused by a bacterial infection and usually treated by antibiotics.

Myocarditis is inflammation of the heart muscles. The exact cause of Myocarditis is unknown. Treatment includes medications and physiotherapy.

Pericarditis always makes me think of Pterodactyls for some reason. But it's got nothing to do with flying dinosaurs. Pericarditis is inflammation of the lining of a sac that contains the heart. There are various causes of Pericarditis including:

❖ Bacterial or viral infection, including COVID-19.

❖ Inflammatory conditions such as Rheumatoid Arthritis (see p54).

❖ Diseases such as cancer (see p119-120), underactive thyroid (see p82-86) and acute kidney failure (see p104-105).

❖ Significant injury or trauma to the chest.

❖ Some medications and vaccines.

Myocardial Infarction (Heart Attack) (MI) is a sudden blockage of the blood supply to the heart in most cases caused by a blood clot. An MI is a medical emergency and life saving immediate treatment is required.

An MI can lead to cell death (medical term: Necrosis) of the heart muscle, due to the lack of blood supply. This cell death is permanent and can result in a damaged heart that can't function properly. The death of too many cells can result in a cardiac arrest and death.

The blood clots that cause MIs are usually caused by Coronary Heart Disease (CHD) (see below for CHD information) or a lack of oxygen in the blood (medical term: Hypoxia).

MIs can't be prevented, but the risk of experiencing MIs can be reduced by lifestyle changes and medications.

Symptoms of an MI include:
* ❖ Chest pain **(individuals with diabetes don't always have chest pain)**.

* ❖ Shortness of breath.

* ❖ Feeling dizzy.

* ❖ Sweating.

* ❖ Feeling sick (medical term: Nausea) and vomiting.

* ❖ Anxiety

* ❖ Jaw or back pain.

* ❖ Coughing and a wheeze.

* ❖ Late symptoms include becoming unconscious and unresponsive and an individual may require CPR.

Symptoms vary from individual to individual and can vary from MI to MI. An individual may have just some of the symptoms listed above, but not necessarily all of them.

Treatments include:
* ❖ Medications to breakdown the blood clot and reduce the risk of further clots.

* ❖ A medication that widens the blood vessels to aid blood flow around the clot.

* ❖ Medications to reduce the blood pressure and pressure on the heart.

* ❖ Painkillers.

* ❖ A surgically implanted Stent - A stent is a short tube inserted to keep the artery open and in some cases to prevent blockage from occuring in the future. This treatment is known as Percutaneous Coronary Intervention (PCI).

* ❖ Various surgical operations with varying aims. The aims of surgery might include: removal of the clot, to create a vessel to bypass the clot, to strengthen the heart/vessels as appropriate.

* ❖ Rehabilitation exercises post MI to build up the strength of the heart.

* ❖ Lifestyle changes post MI to reduce the risk of further MIs.

Cardiogenic & Hypovolemic Shock
Cardiogenic shock is caused by heart problems.

Hypovolemic shock is caused by too little fluid in the cardiovascular system. This can be caused by vessels leaking fluid into the surrounding tissue, or internal or external bleeding usually caused by trauma or injury.

CHD is a disease where fatty substances build up in the arteries of the body, with the potential to cause blockages in the cardiovascular system. It can also be known as Ischaemic Heart Disease or Coronary Artery Disease.

CHD is generally progressive, meaning it gets worse as time progresses. There is no cure for CHD, but there are a range of lifestyle changes and medications that can be used to treat it and prevent further deterioration.

People most at risk of CHD are those with high blood pressure, high cholesterol, long term chronic diseases such as diabetes, those with a family history of CHD, those that are overweight and physically underactive and people who smoke or have smoked in the past.

Chest pain and being short of breath are the two main symptoms of CHD. CHD can lead to other heart conditions such as MIs (heart attacks), Angina and even heart failure (see below for more details of heart failure).

Treatments for CHD include lifestyle changes and medications. All with the aim of slowing CHD, reducing the risks of developing other conditions and treating symptoms.

Heavy alcohol use can cause both irregular heart beat (medical term: Arrhythmia) and Cardiomyopathy (see above). The risk of these conditions can be minimised by reducing alcohol consumption.

Heart Failure is a chronic long term disease which gets worse as time progresses. There is no cure and is caused by the heart becoming too weak to efficiently circulate the blood supply around the body. As heart failure is essentially about the heart struggling to cope, the symptoms are wide ranging and are likely to include:
  ❖ Extreme fatigue.

  ❖ Swollen ankles and feet, caused by a buildup of fluid in them (medical term: Oedema).

  ❖ Being short of breath, particularly when active like walking, even short distances.

❖ Feeling lightheaded.

❖ Possible falls due to a sudden drop of blood pressure on standing.

❖ Weight gain or loss.

❖ Sometimes confusion.

❖ A fast pulse rate.

❖ An irregular heartbeat and palpitations.

Treatments are lifestyle changes, medications and surgically implanted devices (such as a pacemaker).

A Note on Intravenous Drug Users (IVDU) & The Heart
Individuals who inject drugs intravenously are at greater risk of pericarditis (see above) and also infections of valves of the heart. Both are treated with intravenous antibiotics.

DVT (Deep Vein Thrombosis) is a blood clot. They most commonly occur in the leg, but can also occur in arms and the abdominal area. The exact cause of a DVT blood clot is unknown.

There are factors that can increase the risk of an individual getting a DVT (such as being immobile, smoking and obesity). But anyone can get a DVT, including someone that has never smoked and is otherwise fit and well.

Symptoms of a DVT include swelling and redness to the affected area (e.g. leg), it may feel warm to the touch and tenderness/pain to touch. Medications aimed at thinning the blood (such as Warfarin) are prescribed, along with surgery to remove the clot.

Haemophilia is a condition where an individual has lower levels of platelets than other people. It is a genetically inherited condition. Most people are aware if there is a family history of Haemophilia, but some are not.

Haemophilia is graded as mild, moderate or severe. Symptoms of Haemophilia include sudden nosebleeds, bleeding gums and sometimes internal bleeding of joints and muscles.

Haemophilia is treated with medications (injections to increase clotting factors that can be self-administered at home). In cases of trauma or injury, an individual with Haemophilia may require blood transfusions. These blood transfusions may be full or specific blood products (such as platelets) and surgery may be required to stop internal bleeding.

Sickle Cell is a genetically inherited condition which affects the red blood cells. In sickle cell, the red blood cells that the body creates are misshapen and don't live as long as healthy ones. It is more prevalent in people with an African or Caribbean family heritage.

Sickle Cell's symptoms include:
- ❖ Sickle Cell Crises - Episodes of severe pain caused by blood vessels becoming blocked.

- ❖ Regularly acquiring infections (both bacterial and viral).

- ❖ Low levels of Haemoglobin (a protein in red blood cells which binds oxygen to it). An interesting fact about Haemoglobin: Each red blood cell contains several hundred million of these proteins.

- ❖ Delayed growth or development.

- ❖ Liver problems, including jaundice.

- ❖ Painful joints and bones.

- ❖ Legs ulcers.

- Strokes (see p15).

- Swelling of the Spleen (see p57).

- Pulmonary Hypertension (see below).

- Bladder and Kidney problems (see p102-106).

Treatments for sickle cell depend on the symptoms being experienced by an individual with sickle cell. But treatments include pain management, use of heat pads on affected areas and distraction therapy. Daily antibiotics to prevent bacterial infections. Keeping up-to-date with vaccinations, including seasonal vaccinations such as for the Flu. Sometimes surgery to remove the gallbladder.

In rare cases people with sickle cell may be offered stem cell or bone marrow transplants. These are only offered in very rare cases due to the significant risks surrounding the procedures.

Pulmonary Hypertension is a high blood pressure in the arteries that supply blood to the lungs. There are number of causes of Pulmonary Hypertension including:
- Portal Hypertension - A high blood pressure of the vein that supplies blood to the liver.

- Birth Defects - Such as a hole in the heart.

- Certain Medications.

- Human Immunodeficiency Virus (HIV) (see below).

- Thyroid Malfunctions (see p82-86).

- Sickle cell disease (see above) or any condition that affects haemoglobin levels.

- Lung Cancer (see p119-120).

- Chronic Kidney Disease (see P106).

Pulmonary Hypertension is also linked to COPD (see p64-66), Sleep Apnea (see p62-63) and previous blood clots. However how these conditions relate to Pulmonary Hypertension is currently a topic of some debate.

There is no cure for Pulmonary Hypertension, treatment usually focuses on treating the underlying condition causing Pulmonary Hypertension. This may include medications and occasionally surgery.

Sudden Arrhythmic Death Syndrome (SADS) is a condition in which an irregular heart beat causes a cardiac arrest and usually sadly results in death. It usually affects younger people, but can affect anyone of any age. The exact cause of SADS is often unknown, even after autopsy. SADS can sometimes run in families, suggesting that in some cases there could be a genetic link.

There is often no way of detecting SADS in advance of cardiac arrest, so the only treatment is to try and revive the individual using resuscitation methods.

Thalassaemia is an umbrella term for a group of genetic conditions which affect haemoglobin levels. In thalassaemia haemoglobin levels are abnormally low or high.

Some people with thalassaemia can have it from birth, whereas others can develop the condition at any point in their life. Thalassaemia affects people with a Mediterranean (including Italy, Greece & Cyprus), Asian (including India, Pakistan, Bangladesh & China) or Middle Eastern heritage.

Symptoms of thalassaemia depend on the type, but can include Low iron levels (medical term: Anaemia) or having too much iron in the body. Too much iron in the body can cause:

❖ Cardiomyopathy, irregular heartbeat and heart failure.

❖ Thyroid problems, see p82-86 for further details.

❖ Diabetes, see P48-52 for further details.

❖ Damage to the liver, including permanent cirrhosis. This can lead to presentations with jaundice.

❖ Low hormone levels in both males (testosterone) and female (oestrogen).

❖ Late puberty and reduced fertility.

❖ Gallbladder problems including inflammation and gallstones.

❖ Problems with bone growth, usually evident by enlarged forehead or cheeks and osteoporosis.

Thalassaemia can be cured with stem cell or bone marrow transplants, however these are rarely undertaken due to the significant risks involved with the procedures.

Treatment for Anaemia is injections of Vitamin B12 (iron) and regular blood transfusions. Treatment for too much iron in the body is medications to help the body remove excess iron. Treatments for those with high iron levels, also include treating any other conditions that develop as a result of this.

Human Immunodeficiency Virus (HIV) is a blood borne virus (BBV) that is usually spread by having unprotected sex or by sharing injecting equipment with someone that has HIV. It can also be spread from mother to baby during pregnancy, during the birthing process or through breastfeeding.

HIV is not the only BBV, another common one is Hepatitis C. Hepatitis C is covered on p100-101, as it made sense to put all types of Hepatitis together and in the chapter that covers the liver.

HIV attacks and weakens the immune system, leaving an individual at significant risk of other bacterial and viral infections.

Acquired Immune Deficiency Syndrome (AIDS) is a late stage of HIV and is when the immune system has been compromised to a level that it is considered life threatening. Usually someone in the AIDS stage will have another disease such as TB (see p63-64), pneumonia (see p65-66) or cancer (see p119).

Usually after an individual has been infected with HIV they will have flu-like symptoms within 2-6 weeks. These symptoms usually last 1-2 weeks, but can sometimes last longer. After this there can be no symptoms of HIV for years (medical term: Asymptomatic).

There isn't a cure for HIV, but there are medications that can reduce the HIV viral load to undetectable levels.

There is also Post-Exposure Prophylaxis (PEP) emergency treatment available for anyone that feels they may have been exposed to the HIV virus. PEP must be started within 72 hours of exposure and aims to prevent HIV from infecting the individual.

Abdominal Aortic Aneurysm (AAA) is swelling to the aortic artery that supplies the abdominal area. AAA becomes a problem if it bursts (medical term: ruptures) leading to a massive amount of blood loss and sadly usually death.

Joke: How did they discover that he wasn't a real Doctor?
By his good handwriting.

Chapter 9 - The Endocrine System

The endocrine system is made up of organs that produce hormones in the human body. A hormone is essentially a chemical messenger.

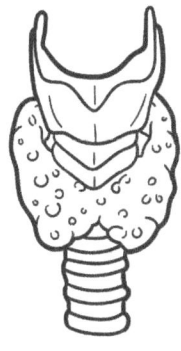

The Thyroid is a gland that produces hormones that help keep the human body functioning normally (medical term: Homeostasis).

The Thyroid is located in the neck of the human body. The Thyroid is not the only producer of hormones, but it is an important one. And it can malfunction.

The Thyroid.

The Thyroid can malfunction by being overactive (medical term: Hyperthyroidism or Thyrotoxicosis) or underactive (medical term: Hypothyroidism).

An overactive thyroid can be caused by Graves' Disease (see below), lumps on the thyroid (called nodules), some medications used to treat other conditions, a multiple or molar pregnancy, a non-cancerous growth in the pituitary gland, a bacterial or viral infection and on rare occasions cancer in the Thyroid.

The symptoms of an overactive Thyroid include:

❖ Anxiety or irritability.

❖ Mood swings.

❖ A lump in the neck.

❖ Thyroiditis is inflammation of the Thyroid gland. It can sometimes be caused by a bacterial infection that will require antibiotics to treat it or a virus which usually resolves without treatment in 7-10 days or one of the causes below.

❖ A feeling of having too much energy - yet feeling tired or exhausted all the time.

❖ Palpitations or an irregular heart beat.

❖ Difficulty sleeping (medical term: Insomnia).

❖ Muscle weakness, twitching or trembling.

❖ Extreme thirst/increased fluid intake/increased peeing (medica term: Urination).

❖ Hives on the skin, causing itchiness.

❖ Hair loss (Alopecia, see p32-33 for other causes).

❖ Increased appetite and dietary intake, yet losing weight.

❖ Loose stools.

❖ Loss of interest in or desire to have sex.

As these symptoms persist sometimes over weeks or months, they can have a real impact on an individual's mental health and quality of life.

Graves' Disease is an autoimmune condition in which white blood cells mistake cells in the thyroid that regulate the production and release of hormones as foreign and attack them. This leads to an overactive thyroid.

Lumps (called nodules) can develop that also have hormone producing cells in them resulting in too much of the hormones that the thyroid produces in the human body.

Some medications can cause an overactive thyroid. Iodine is a mineral found in some foods and medications. Iodine is required by the thyroid to make hormones, but too much iodine in the body causes the thyroid to become overactive. The usual treatment in the case of too much iodine caused by medication is to discontinue or change the medication. This usually solves the problem, although it can take several months before hormone levels reduce and return to normal.

A multiple pregnancy is when a female is pregnant with two or more unborn babies at the same time and can cause an overactive thyroid.

As can a molar pregnancy. A molar pregnancy is rare and is an abnormal growth of the embryo cells during early pregnancy. Sadly, there is no cure or treatments for a molar pregnancy and it results in miscarriage.

It is essential that an overactive thyroid is identified and treated during pregnancy to prevent complications during the pregnancy or during labour.

Sometimes an overactive thyroid can be the result of a non-cancerous growth in the pituitary gland. The pituitary gland is located in the very centre of the brain and is known as the 'master gland.' It communicates with all the other hormone producing glands in the human body instructing them on how to operate. When there is pressure on the pituitary gland, it can't function normally and this results in overactivity in the thyroid. For more details about the pituitary gland see below.

Treatments for an overactive Thyroid depend on the underlying cause, but may include medications (or changing medications for other conditions) - it should be noted that some of these medications take up to 12-18 months to be effective, sometimes radiotherapy (radioactive iodine treatment) and in some cases surgery.

An underactive Thyroid is when the gland doesn't produce enough hormones. An underactive thyroid usually occurs after the immune system attacks the hormone producing cells in the thyroid and it has been overactive. The thyroid can also become underactive due to damage occurring during treatments for an overactive thyroid (see above) and rarely due to cancer in the thyroid.

An underactive thyroid can have the following symptoms:

❖ Fatigue.

❖ Depression (see p10-11 for more information).

❖ Weight gain.

❖ A feeling that thoughts and actions have become much slower than normal.

❖ Being unable to open bowels or problems having bowel movements (medical term: Constipation).

❖ Pain/Tingling/Numbness to hands (medical term: Carpal Tunnel Syndrome).

❖ Increased and regular muscle aches, pains and cramps.

❖ Hearing loss (see p23-26 for more details on causes of hearing loss). This is generally a symptom that develops after living with an underactive thyroid for some time without treatment.

❖ Loss of interest in or desire to have sex.

❖ Specific to females who are reproductively active: Heavier periods, with the risk that they also become irregular.

❖ Specific to children: delayed growth and in reaching developmental milestones.

❖ Specific to adolescents: May start puberty earlier than expected.

❖ Specific to older people: May develop problems with memory.

There is no cure for an underactive thyroid. However treatment is straightforward with hormone replacement therapy, a daily tablet containing the hormones your thyroid used to produce. It is accompanied by regular blood tests to check that the dose is strong enough and that the individual with an underactive thyroid has the correct levels of hormones in their blood.

Treatment usually resolves the symptoms above, but once the hormone levels are correct, if any symptoms persist tests and investigations to identify other causes of the symptoms may be undertaken. Along with other medications or treatments to treat the ongoing symptoms.

The pituitary and pineal glands are located in the brain. The pituitary gland releases hormones responsible for growth and development, metabolism, reproduction, the body's response to stress and trauma, lactation and childbirth (in females) and water/salt balance. The pituitary gland malfunctioning is associated with a number of conditions. The pituitary gland can malfunction by:

❖ A non-cancerous growth influencing normal operation (medical term: Pituitary Adenomas) - Symptoms can include loss of vision, headaches, weight gain, changes in bone structures (particularly face & hands), changes to menstrual cycle in females, erectile dysfunction in males. Surgery is the usual treatment, medications and sometimes radiotherapy.

❖ The pituitary gland not producing or not producing one or more hormones (medical term: Hypopituitarism). Symptoms depend on which hormones are affected but can include: delayed growth and development, late puberty and fertility. Treatment is hormone replacement medications.

❖ The pituitary gland producing too much of a hormone or hormones (medical term: Hyperpituitarism). Symptoms can include enlarged hands/feet and sometimes organs, rarely Gigantism (a condition in which an individual is incredibly tall) and the production of too much cortisol (the stress hormone).

The pineal gland releases the hormone melatonin. There are three things that can go wrong with this gland:

* ❖ Calcification of the pineal gland - As people get older some calcification of the gland can occur and is normal. However, too much calcification can cause the gland not to be able to function normally.

* ❖ Injury or trauma to the pineal gland usually caused by a significant head injury or raised intracranial pressure.

* ❖ Rarely a cancerous brain tumour can cause the pineal gland to malfunction.

Symptoms of a problem with the pineal gland can include seizures, issues with memory, confusion, headaches, nausea/vomiting and changes to vision. Some people may only get some of these symptoms. Treatment depends on the cause but will usually include medications, surgery and sometimes radiotherapy.

The adrenal glands are located at the top of the kidneys and responsible for the release of adrenaline and noradrenaline. Addison's Disease (also known as medical term: Hypoadrenalism) is low levels of adrenaline in the body. Addison's disease is caused by a faulty immune system attacking the adrenaline producing cells in the glands. It can run in families suggesting a genetic link, but TB can also damage the adrenal glands.

Symptoms of Addison's disease include extreme fatigue, loss of appetite with or without weight loss, lowered blood pressure, nausea/vomiting, muscle weakness and cramps, abdominal pain, depression, low levels of energy & motivation, increased thirst with increased frequency of urination, a high temperature, irregular periods in females, late puberty and sometimes episodes of low blood sugar.

People with Addison's disease can have crisis episodes where levels of adrenaline become so low that it becomes life threatening. Symptoms of an Addison's crisis include:

* ❖ Dehydration.

❖ Sweating.

❖ Skin becoming pale and clammy.

❖ Low blood pressure with dizziness and vasovagal episodes (fainting).

❖ Vomiting and diarrhoea.

❖ Abdominal pain.

❖ Extreme fatigue and a reduced level of consciousness.

An Addison's crisis can be life threatening and immediate medical treatment should be sought, otherwise it can result in death.

There is no cure for Addison's disease. Treatments for Addison's include long term antibiotics, steroids, as well as other medications to relieve or manage symptoms.

Joke: What is the difference between a hormone and a vitamin?
I never made a vitamin.

Chapter 10 -The Gastrointestinal System

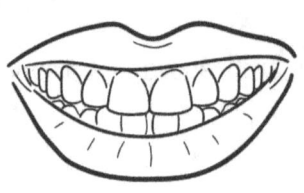

Teeth

The gastrointestinal system is made up of the teeth, the tongue, the mouth, the oesophagus, the stomach, the gut (large and small intestines), the bowel, the gallbladder, the pancreas and the liver.

This is probably the longest chapter in the book, this is due to the sheer number of ways the gastrointestinal system can go wrong.

Let's begin with the teeth.

Tooth decay is when a hole gradually develops in one or more teeth. It is thought to be caused by a combination of poor oral hygiene (not regularly brushing teeth with fluoride toothpaste) and eating too many foods high in sugar.

Symptoms of tooth decay can include: toothache, a sharp pain when eating something cold/very hot and visible

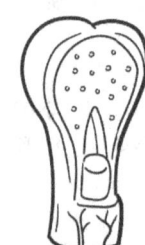

The Inside of a Tooth.

white/brown/black spots on teeth. Sometimes a dental abscess or repeat abscesses can indicate tooth decay (see p119 for more details on abscesses).

There is no cure for tooth decay. Depending on what stage of tooth decay has occurred will depend on the treatment. A filling (filling the hole) may be an option, however if decay has reached the soft tissue a root canal treatment will be required. Sometimes decay has become so bad that a tooth or teeth needs to be removed (medical term: extraction).

A Note On: Orthodontic Treatment
In approximately one third of people teeth don't grow as they

should. The cause of this is unknown.

Signs that teeth aren't growing as they should include an uneven bite, teeth not growing straight/being crooked, too many teeth in the mouth - causing teeth to sometimes overlap and gaps between teeth.

In these cases Orthodontic treatment may be required. This treatment involves fitting a brace/retainer/both to teeth to straighten them and ensure that they grow as they should.

Sensitive teeth are a warning sign that the enamel on a tooth or teeth has been damaged. Symptoms of sensitive teeth include sensitivity or pain when eating or drinking something very hot/very cold/very sweet and discomfort/pain when biting down onto something.

Sensitive teeth are usually reversible by regularly brushing with a sensitive toothpaste. However if sensitive teeth don't improve or get worse see a Dentist. This is because the longer you leave sensitive teeth, the worse the damage could be and the more discomfort/pain experienced.

The cause of Teeth Grinding (medical term: Bruxism) is sometimes unknown but is often linked to:
  ❖ Mental Illnesses such as anxiety.
  ❖ Stress either Acute or Chronic.
  ❖ Sleep Apnoea (see p62-63).
  ❖ Certain medications including common antidepressants.
  ❖ Alcohol, Smoking and Drug Use.

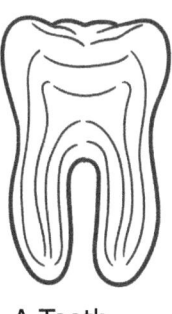

A Tooth.

Symptoms of Teeth Grinding include waking up with sore teeth, jaw pain, shoulder/neck/face pain, headaches, earaches and disturbed sleep.

There is no cure for teeth grinding, but depending on the cause there are treatments. Treating the underlying cause of teeth grinding usually resolves it. Use of a mouth guard will protect the teeth from becoming damaged due to the grinding of teeth.

Gum Disease is caused by a buildup of plaque on the teeth and gums. Symptoms include swollen/sore gums, regular bleeding when brushing teeth, teeth becoming loose and falling out, bad taste in mouth and bad breath.

There is no cure for Gum Disease but there are treatments which include information and advice (including going Smoke-Free), medications and occasional surgery.

The cause of Mouth Ulcers varies. Causes include:

❖ Injury to your gums, inside of cheeks including burns from hot diet and fluids.

❖ Badly fitting braces/retainers/dentures with the mouth ulcer caused by repeated rubbing on gums/insides of mouth.

❖ Stress and anxiety.

❖ Genetics are sometimes thought to play a role as recurrent mouth ulcers run in families.

❖ Hormonal changes such as when puberty starts and in females during pregnancy.

❖ Thiamine (Vitamin B12) or iron deficiency.

❖ Some medicines can trigger mouth ulcers.

Mouth Ulcers generally resolve on their own within 1-2 weeks. Advice should be sought from a Dentist if a mouth ulcer is still present after 3 weeks or mouth ulcers are recurring. As always, treating the underlying cause of mouth ulcers is key to preventing future reoccurrences.

Halitosis (medical term) or bad breath is caused by poor oral hygiene. It is treated by the individual not being a *dirty animal*, brushing their teeth/gums/tongue, flossing and using mouthwash.

In all seriousness, persistent bad breath can be a sign of Cancer (see P119-120) and if other symptoms are present medical assessment should be sought out immediately.

Temporomandibular Disorder (TMD) is a malfunction of the jaw. TMD can be caused by teeth grinding (see above), an uneven bite, injury or trauma to the head or face, stress and the joint being worn out by wear and tear. TMD's main symptom is a painful jaw that may radiate to the ears/temples, headaches, clicking/popping noises when the jaw is moved, difficulty fully opening the mouth or the mouth locking once opened.

In most cases of TMD it resolves on its own without any medical treatment. However some people will require stronger painkillers than what is available over the counter and it is usually worth treating the underlying cause of TMD to prevent recurrence.

Tonsillitis can be caused by a viral or bacterial infection that causes the tonsils at the back of the throat to become inflamed.

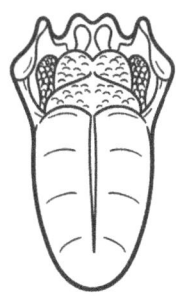

The symptoms of Tonsillitis are a sore/painful throat, a high temperature, headaches, earache and fatigue.

In the case of viral Tonsillitis symptoms usually start to resolve in 3-7 days (it can

Inside of the Mouth & Tongue.

take slightly longer if someone has a weakened or suppressed immune system). Bacterial Tonsillitis may require antibiotics prescribed by a Doctor.

The Adenoids are located at the back of the throat behind the nose. In some children they become enlarged and have to be removed by surgery. They are only removed if they are impacting a child's quality of life. Enlarged Adenoids can cause difficulties in breathing through the nose, can cause sleep apnea (see p62-63), glue ear (see p25-26) and frequent ear/nose/throat infections.

Thrush can affect genitals (of both females and males), but can also affect the mouth. It can also affect armpits, groins and between fingers. For more details about the causes, symptoms and treatments see p109.

Nutcracker Oesophagus (medical term: Achalasia) is a malfunction of the nerves that controls the muscles in the oesophagus (including the lower esophageal sphincter), causing difficulties swallowing and eating food.

The exact cause of Nutcracker Oesophagus is unknown. Symptoms include difficulties eating and drinking (potentially leading to weight loss), chest/abdominal pain, repeated chest infections, nausea/vomiting, drooling, choking, coughing fits and bringing up undigested food.

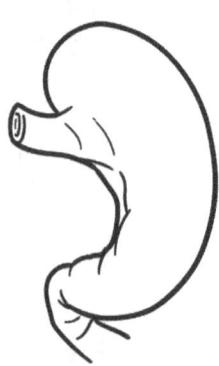

The Stomach.

Gastroesophageal Reflux Disease (GERD) is caused by the sphincter muscle at the top of the stomach becoming weakened and letting stomach acid out into the oesophagus. The exact cause is unknown. GERD causes the following symptoms:

❖ Heartburn.
❖ Acid reflux.
❖ Bloating and bad breath.
❖ Nausea/vomiting.
❖ Pain/difficulty swallowing.
❖ Coughing.
❖ Tooth decay/gum disease (see above).

There is no cure for GERD. But it is treated with lifestyle changes, medications and occasionally surgery.

Gastric/Stomach Ulcers are sores that develop in the lining of the stomach. The causes include bacterial infections or over/regular use of anti-inflammatory medications. Both of which break down the lining of the stomach and leave the stomach being vulnerable to damage and ulceration caused by the stomach acid.

There is some limited evidence that heavy alcohol use and smoking can cause, contribute to the development or prevent the healing of gastric ulcers.

Treatments for gastric ulcers include antibiotic medications, medications that reduce the amount of stomach acid produced (the most common one being Omeprazole), antacid medications and advice around avoiding nonsteroidal anti-inflammatory medications (NSAIDS) such as Ibuprofen or Naproxen.

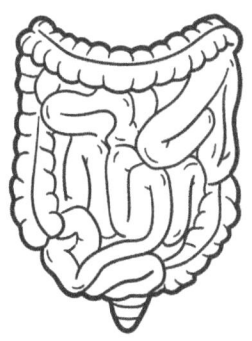

Celiac Disease is a condition in which white blood cells of the immune system attack cells inside the small intestine when a person eats gluten. Although an auto-immue failure, I have opted to include it in this chapter due to symptoms.

Symptoms of celiac disease include:

The Gut.

- ❖ Abdominal pain.
- ❖ Diarrhoea/constipation.
- ❖ Bloating/flatulence.
- ❖ Fatigue.
- ❖ On some occasions: weight loss, fertility issues in females, nerve damage, an unsteady gait and problems with speech.

Treatment for celiac disease involves a lifestyle change in terms of switching to a gluten-free diet.

The cause of Irritable Bowel Syndrome (IBS) is unknown. Symptoms include abdominal pain/stomach cramps, bloating, tiredness, nausea, diarrhoea/constipation and in some cases bowel incontinence. IBS can be painful and unpleasant to experience. Individuals with IBS generally have periods of time being asymptomatic (symptom-free) and episodes or flare ups where symptoms are present.

There is no cure for IBS but there are treatments which are based on the symptoms experienced. These treatments may include lifestyle changes (changes to diet) and medications.

Inflammatory Bowel Disease (IBD) is an umbrella term to describe chronic and long term conditions that affect the bowel. Included under IBD are Crohn's Disease & Ulcerative Colitis.

Crohn's Disease is caused by parts of the gastrointestinal system becoming inflamed. There are a number of theories about the cause of Crohn's disease, but none of these theories have been adequately and scientifically proven. Individuals with Crohn's disease can have constant symptoms or episodic flare ups or both. During a flare up symptoms are more severe.

Symptoms of Crohn's disease include the following:
- ❖ Abdominal pain and cramps that can be agony.

- ❖ Diarrhoea without any other cause.

- ❖ Blood from the bowel during movements or in the faeces afterwards.

- ❖ Fatigue.

- ❖ Weight loss, without trying to lose weight.

- ❖ Sometimes a raised temperature.

- ❖ Patches of red swollen painful skin, usually on the legs, but can occur anywhere on the body.

- ❖ Mouth ulcers (see above).

❖ Anxiety & depression (see p10-11).
There is currently no cure for Crohn's disease and treatments are medications to manage symptoms as required.

Ulcerative Colitis is similar to Crohn's disease. In Ulcerative Colitis the large intestine and rectum (this is where faeces is stored after digestion until an individual opens their bowels) become inflamed. The exact cause is not known but it is thought to be an autoimmune system malfunction.

Ulcerative Colitis symptoms are the same as the symptoms of Crohn's disease. As with Crohn's disease there is currently no cure for Ulcerative Colitis and the treatments available help to manage symptoms.

Joke: A man went to hospital with 4 plastic horses up his rectum. The doctors described his condition as stable.

A Note on Bowel Incontinence
Bowel Incontinence can have a number of causes including IBS, IBD, severe piles (see below) and lower nerve damage. Although Bowel Incontinence is more a symptom than a condition, it is worth noting here due to the impact it can have on those individuals affected.

Symptoms of Bowel Incontinence include:
❖ Having a sudden uncontrollable urge to go to the toilet.
❖ Opening bowels without being aware of it.
❖ Bowels can open everyday or on episodic occasions.
❖ Leaking of faeces when unexpected.
❖ Affects daily living including socialisation.
❖ Anxiety and depression.

Treatments for Bowel Incontinence involve identifying and treating any underlying condition, changes to lifestyle (in particular diet and exercise routines), incontinence products, medication/changes to medication, pelvic floor exercises (in females), bowel retraining and occasionally surgery.

Diverticulitis is a bacterial infection in the large intestine. Symptoms include:

❖ Abdominal pain, typically worse on the left side of an individual.

❖ A high temperature with or without sweating.

❖ Diarrhoea or an increased frequency of needing to open bowels.

Diverticulitis is treated with oral or intravenous antibiotics and painkiller medications.

Piles (medical term: Haemorrhoids) are swollen blood vessels inside and around an individual's bottom (medical term: Anus). Piles are caused by any sort of straining. This can include lifting something heavy, coughing fits and constipation/diarrhoea.

Piles can sometimes resolve on their own. If they do not, therapies at hospital can help, medications (such as painkillers and topical creams) and occasionally surgery can all treat piles.

The gallbladder stores bile created by the liver and releases it into the intestines. Like any organ the gallbladder can malfunction. One of the ways the gallbladder can malfunction is through the creation of gallstones.

Gallstones are theorised to be caused by an imbalance in the chemicals in the gallbladder. Gallstones are common and often give no symptoms. But when they do they cause constant severe pain, in some cases jaundice and a high temperature. Treatment for gallstones is medications to manage pain (painkillers), sometimes medications to break down the gallstones and sometimes surgical removal of the gallbladder.

Inflammation of the gallbladder (medical term: Cholecystitis) is usually acute (sudden onset) and can be caused by the cystic duct (the opening to the gallbladder) becomes blocked by a gallstone or substance called biliary sludge. In around 5% of cases the cause of inflammation of the gallbladder is unknown. The following symptoms are signs of an inflamed gallbladder:

❖ Persistent abdominal pain, that doesn't go away.

❖ Nausea/vomiting.

❖ A high temperature, along with sweating.

❖ Jaundice.

❖ A lump in the abdominal area that is tender/painful.

Medical assessment and treatment should always be sought for cases of suspected Cholecystitis. Treatment involves fasting (Nil By Mouth), intravenous fluids, painkillers, potentially intravenous antibiotics if there is a bacterial infection and possibly surgery to remove the gallbladder.

Colorectal Polyps are polyps that develop in the large intestine or rectum. The cause is thought to be abnormal cell growth caused by faulty genetics. They are non-cancerous growths and are only usually removed if causing symptoms. For most individuals they are asymptomatic and require no treatment.

Symptoms of colorectal polyps include rectal bleeding (a small amount of blood being passed when opening bowels), abdominal pain and diarrhoea/constipation (without other causes identified).

Colorectal polyps that do require treatment can usually be treated by a colonoscopy (a camera up the anus that can identify, burn off and cauterise the resulting wound). On exceptionally rare occasions part of the large intestine may need to be surgically removed.

The pancreas creates the hormone insulin as part of the digestive process. Pancreatitis is inflammation of the pancreas. Pancreatitis can be acute (sudden onset) or chronic.

Acute Pancreatitis can be caused by:

- ❖ A bacterial or viral infection.

- ❖ Gallstones (see above).

- ❖ Drinking too much alcohol, usually (but not always) daily drinking of large quantities.

- ❖ High levels of Calcium in the blood (see Electrolyte imbalances on p69 for more details).

- ❖ White blood cells attacking the pancreas (known as Autoimmune Pancreatitis).

Symptoms of acute pancreatitis include abdominal pain, a high temperature, nausea/vomiting, jaundice and increased heart/breathing rates.

Pancreatitis requires hospital admission for intravenous fluids and other medications (including steroids, antibiotics, painkillers, etc.). It usually resolves in around a week with medical treatments/care.

Chronic pancreatitis is where the pancreas has become permanently damaged and has episodic flare ups with the same symptoms as acute pancreatitis and treatments to resolve (see above). If an individual has more than one episode of pancreatitis they have chronic pancreatitis.

The liver filters the blood removing toxins and other harmful substances from the bloodstream.

Portal Hypertension is a high blood pressure in the liver, stopping the liver from functioning effectively. It is usually caused by excessive alcohol consumption but can occasionally be due to Hepatitis (see below).

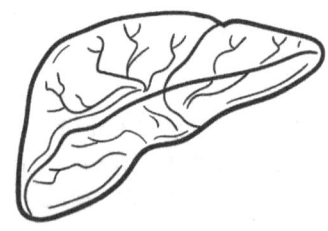

The Liver

Treatments for portal hypertension include medications and endoscopic treatments. On some occasions liver transplant may be offered, but there is a waiting list for liver transplant, an individual must be alcohol-free and this comes with long term immunosuppressant medications.

Hepatitis is inflammation of the liver. Here are the five main types:

Type	Causes & Symptoms
A	Hepatitis A is caused by food contaminated by microscopic particles of faeces. It can be prevented by good hand hygiene. Symptoms of Hepatitis A are very mild and usually self-resolve. Most individuals who get Hepatitis A put it down to a bad case of food poisoning, the flu or other illness. There is a vaccine as a preventative measure.
B	Hepatitis B is caused by blood to blood contact and is usually caused by sex with an infected individual or sharing injecting equipment in the case of injecting drugs intravenously (IVDU). Sometimes it can be spread from mother to baby during labour. Symptoms of this form of Hepatitis include a temperature, fatigue, nausea/vomiting and jaundice. Treatment includes medications and symptom management. There is a vaccine as a preventative measure.
C	Hepatitis C is caused by blood to blood contact and is usually caused by sex with an infected individual or sharing injecting equipment in the case of IVDUs. Symptoms of Hepatitis C include the following:

	❖ Abdominal pain. ❖ Nausea/vomiting. ❖ Fatigue. ❖ A high temperature. ❖ Difficulty concentrating. ❖ Anxiety and depression (see p10-11). ❖ Itchy skin. ❖ Bloating. Medications can treat Hepatitis C and sometimes these help the body clear the virus. Other times it becomes chronic and can lead to liver failure. On-going medication treatments help minimise this risk. There is a vaccine as a preventative measure.
D	Hepatitis D needs Hepatitis B in the body in order to survive. It is caused by blood to blood contact and is usually caused by sex with an infected individual or sharing injecting equipment in the case of IVDUs. Symptoms and treatments are similar to other types of Hepatitis (see above).
E	Hepatitis E is caused by contaminated or undercooked foods. Most people think they have food poisoning or other illness and it doesn't require medical treatment.

<u>What is Jaundice?</u>
Jaundice is the yellowing of the skin and whites of the eyes. Put simply, Jaundice is toxins that the liver is unable to process due to some impairment that is put into other tissues around the body. It always requires urgent medical attention.

Liver disease comes in stages and can have a number of causes. For more details, check out The British Liver Trust website for more information. Details of this disease have been deliberately excluded from this book as the cause is usually alcohol-related.

Chapter 11 - The Urinary System

The urinary system is made up of the bladder, two Kidneys and tubes from the kidneys to the bladder (medical term: Ureters).

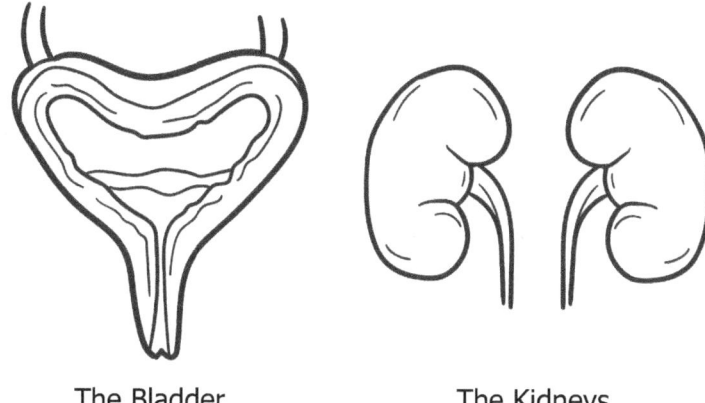

The Bladder   The Kidneys.

Bladder and Kidney Stones are both malfunctions of the urinary system. Bladder stones are caused by minerals in the bladder that buildup to become stones when the bladder isn't fully emptied on a regular basis. Kidney stones are caused by a buildup of certain chemicals in the body.

Symptoms of bladder stones include passing of dark coloured urine, pain when urinating, increased frequency of urination, blood in the urine and severe lower abdominal pain/pain around the genitals area.

Symptoms of kidney stones include severe pain in the lower abdomen/genitals area (that may be constant or come and go), a high temperature (medical term: Hyperpyrexia), nausea/vomiting, blood in urine and infections in the bladder.

Surgery can be completed to remove both bladder and larger kidney stones. Medications are also used to treat symptoms including anti-sickness (medical term: Antiemetics) drugs, anti-inflammatory drugs (such as Ibuprofen) and painkillers.

Paruresis is the fear of urinating and or opening bowels. It is sometimes called shy bladder syndrome or psychogenic urinary retention.

People with paruresis have difficulty urinating and may actively avoid doing so. They may have fear about being too far from toilets, fear of using public toilets or fear that people may be watching or listening to them on the toilet. Due to the condition being psychological rather than physiological in nature, individuals with Paruresis are reluctant to get help and often struggle alone for years.

There is a lack of specialist services for paruresis. But often counselling, CBT and lifestyle changes can help. The first step for an individual with paruresis would be to speak to their GP and to get a referral to Community Mental Health Services. In terms of what can be done to support a patient in a Ward/Department setting you can:

- ❖ Reassure the patient that toilets are safe, clean and private spaces.

- ❖ Monitor both urinary and bowel output. It is also useful to record dietary intake and keep a fluid balance.

- ❖ Make the patient aware of potential consequences and possible necessary treatments involved if they don't urinate/open their bowels.

- ❖ Ask: Do you have a problem or fear using our toilets?

- ❖ Ask: Is there anything we can do to support you in urinating/opening bowels during your stay?

Urinary incontinence is uncontrolled urination. There are four different types including:

1. Stress Incontinence - Caused by the bladder being under stress (for example when someone urinates when they laugh, cough or sneeze). Examples of when this is likely to occur:
   - Damage during childbirth (in females).
   - Additional pressure on the bladder caused by pregnancy (in females) or by being overweight (in both genders).
   - Damage to the bladder during surgery for other reasons.
   - Some medications.
   - Some very rare conditions.

2. Urgency Incontinence - Caused by the urgent and sudden need to urinate or just afterwards.
- Not drinking enough fluids or drinking too much caffeine/alcohol.
- Urinary system bacterial infections.
- Constipation.
- Some neurological conditions.
- Some medications.

3. Overflow Incontinence - Caused by the bladder being too full due to not going or being able to go to the toilet (medical term: urinary retention).
- An enlarged prostate (see p110).
- Bladder stones (see above).
- Constipation.

4. Total Incontinence - Caused by the bladder not being able to retain any urine at all. Symptoms of this include constant dribbling/flow of urine.
- A problem with the bladder from birth.
- An injury/trauma to the spinal cord.
- A bladder fistula, which is a hole between the bladder and a nearby area such as the Vagina in females.

Symptoms of Urinary incontinence are above and depend on the type. Treatments depend on the underlying cause and type of incontinence but may include lifestyle changes, medications and on some occasions surgery.

Acute Kidney Injury (AKI) is a sudden stopping or deterioration of the functioning of the kidneys. AKI is sometimes the result of another disease/illness, including conditions/illnesses that affect the amount of blood circulating in the cardiovascular system and therefore the amount of blood reaching the kidneys.

AKI should be considered in anyone dehydrated due to vomiting/diarrhoea, with heart failure (see p75-76), liver failure or Sepsis (see p121).

Symptoms of AKI include nausea/vomiting, dehydration, confusion, diarrhoea, reduced urine output and drowsiness/reduction in consciousness (late symptom).

Treatments for AKI include intravenous fluids, antibiotics (in the case of bacterial infection), stopping certain medications that may make the condition AKI worse and catheterisation to monitor output closely. Along with treating the underlying condition/illnesses causing AKi. In rare cases Dialysis may be required to filter the blood.

Damage to the tiny filters in the kidneys that filter the blood (medical term: Glomerulonephritis) is often caused by the immune system attacking these filters. It is usually an indicator of Lupus (see p52-53), Hepatitis B/C (see p100-101), HIV (see p80-81) or endocarditis (see p72). Mild cases don't cause any symptoms, however more severe cases can cause the following symptoms:

❖ Rashes.

❖ Abdominal/joint pain.

❖ Increased frequency of urination.

❖ A high temperature (above 37.5°C).

❖ Shortness of breath.

❖ Jaundice (yellowing of the skin and whites of the eyes - caused by a buildup of toxins in tissues around the body).

❖ Tiredness with or without weight loss.

Treatment for Glomerulonephritis involves treating the underlying condition causing it. This may include medications (including antibiotics, Intravenous fluids, steroids, medicines to increase frequency of bowel movements & painkillers).

Alport Syndrome (AS) is caused by genetics inherited from biological parents. Symptoms include blood & protein in the urine, high blood pressure, hearing loss starts at around 10 years old and problems with eyes.

AS treatments depend on symptoms experienced but may include medications, remaining hydrated, lifestyle changes, hearing aids and glasses/laser eye surgery.

Chronic Kidney Disease (CKD) is a long term condition where the kidneys don't fully function. CKD is caused by:

❖ High Blood Pressure/High Cholesterol.

❖ Diabetes (see p48-59).

❖ Kidney Infections or Inflammation (including Glomerulonephritis, see above).

❖ Kidney Stones (see above) / Enlarged Prostate (see p110).

❖ Long term use of some medications, the risks of this should be discussed with the individual prior to starting them on these medications on a long term basis.

❖ Autosomal Dominant Polycystic Kidney Disease (ADPKD) (see below).

Treatment options include lifestyle changes, medications (such as those to treat high blood pressure and statins to treat high cholesterol), dialysis and sometimes a Kidney transplant.

Autosomal Dominant Polycystic Kidney Disease (ADPKD) is an inherited condition where cysts develop in the kidneys. Although individuals have ADPKD from birth, it doesn't start to cause kidney problems until around the age of 30-40 years old, once the cysts are big enough to impair kidney functioning.

When ADPKD affects kidney functioning symptoms include: blood in urine (medical term: Haematuria), abdominal pain, high blood pressure and urinary infections.

Treatment for ADPKD involves medication to slow the growth of the cysts, symptom management medications (such as painkillers, antibiotics) and very occasionally surgical interventions.

Chapter 12 - The Male Reproductive System

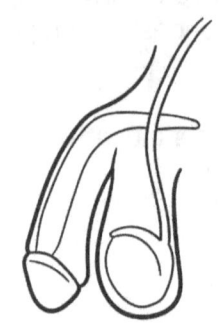

The Penis & Testicles (side view).

The male reproductive system is made up of the penis, testicles and the prostate. Testicles are responsible for producing Sperm Cells. The system is surprisingly simple and as such there are less malfunctions of this system.

The first is Impotence (medical term: Erectile Dysfunction). This is when a male individual is unable to get an erect penis for sexual intercourse to occur or be unable to maintain the erection until climax.

Impotence has several causes including: stress, anxiety/depression, performance anxiety, tiredness, too much alcohol/other depressant drugs, smoking, certain medications (as a side effect), diabetes, high blood pressure/high cholesterol, hormone problems, relationship problems or past sexual assault/abuse.

Treatment will depend on the cause. Lifestyle changes can help such as reducing/stopping smoking/drinking alcohol/other drug use. Eating a good diet, drinking plenty of fluids, getting adequate sleep and exercise can also help. In the case of stress or mental illness, treatment for these conditions can help.

If the cause of impotence is side effects of medications, sometimes medications can be changed for a different one that doesn't have impotence as the side effect. If it is a chronic condition like diabetes, better management of the condition may help.

In the case of past sexual assault or abuse, specialist counselling is recommended to help the individual address their thoughts and feelings about these experiences. Occasionally sessions with a Sex Therapist and/or Couples Counselling can help with impotence.

Low Sex Drive (Loss of Libido) has the same causes and treatments as Impotence.

A Painful Erection (medical term: Priapism) can have several causes including:

❖ Injury (usually through rough sexual intercourse or rough masturbation).

❖ A sickle cell crisis (see p77-78 for more information).

❖ Some medications (including Warfarin, some antidepressants, some medications for high blood pressure and medications for impotence).

❖ Use of Substances (including cocaine & cannabis).

❖ Thalassaemia (see p79-80).

❖ On very rare occasions some forms of cancer (see p119).

Depending on the cause, sometimes a painful erection can be treated at home. These self-treatments include urination, a warm bath/shower, keeping hydrated, going for a walk and taking painkillers.

If a Painful Erection lasts 3-4 hours (1 hour in the case of a sickle cell crisis) medical attention should be sought. Medical treatments include medications, draining blood from the penis and very rarely surgery.

Undescended Testicles are surprisingly common in males at birth. The exact cause of undescended testicles is unknown. But it usually resolves itself by 6 months of age. If the testicles have not resolved by 6 months, treatment involves a surgical procedure to descend the testicles.

Testicular Pain has several causes including:

- ❖ A sudden severe pain is likely to be a Testicular Torsion. A testicular torsion is when the spermatic blood vessel that provides blood to a testicle becomes twisted and cuts off the blood supply to a testicle.

  This leads to cell death (medical term: Necrosis) in the affected testicle. It is a medical emergency.

  Surgery is required to remove the affected testicle, replacing it with a false one. Surprisingly, it doesn't affect the fertility of the male individual.

- ❖ Infections can cause pain. This is usually a bacterial infection and is treated with antibiotics.

- ❖ A hernia can cause testicular pain, see p46 for more details on hernias and their treatments.

- ❖ Injury or trauma - usually through rough sexual intercourse or sports can cause pain. The treatment is usually to wait and see if it heals on its own. Painkiller medications might be given to manage the short term pain.

- ❖ A cyst, which is a build up of non-harmful fluid, can cause testicular pain. Treatments include painkillers and sometimes surgery to drain the cyst.

- ❖ Swollen veins of the testicles can cause pain (medical term: Varicocele). These need treatment as can affect fertility, testosterone levels and can impact on sperm in ejaculation - leading to a condition where no sperm are in ejaculation fluid (medical term: Azoospermia).

Treatments depend on the cause. Both causes and treatments are above.

Thrush (medical term: Candidosis) can occur in both males and females. In males it occurs around the head of the penis. Thrush is caused by a fungal infection and is treated by antifungal topical cream and sometimes an oral tablet.

A Low Sperm Count (medical term: Oligospermia) is usually identified if a hetrosexual couple struggle to conceive a pregnancy. The cause is unknown and there are likely to be multiple different causes. There are treatments that can help with conception in the cases of males with a low sperm count. An interesting fact is that sperm can live inside a female's body for 5-7 days.

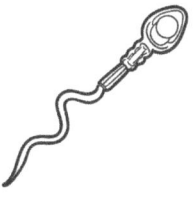

A Sperm Cell.

The prostate's main role is to produce fluid for mixing with sperm cells (produced by the testicles) that are released during ejaculation. The prostate continues to grow as males age and can put pressure on the bladder (medical term: Enlarged Prostate).

An Enlarged Prostate can cause the following symptoms:
* ❖ Difficulty in starting to urinate.

* ❖ A weak urine flow.

* ❖ Feeling strained when peeing.

* ❖ An individual feeling like they can't fully empty their bladder.

* ❖ Incontinence of urine.

* ❖ Dribbling after urination.

* ❖ Urgent and more frequent need to urinate.

* ❖ Waking up in the night to urinate, usually more than once.

Treatments for an Enlarged Prostate include medications and occasionally surgery.

The prostate can also become swollen (medical term: Prostatitis). The cause is sometimes a bacterial infection, although other times the cause is unknown. Symptoms include pain in pelvis/gentiles/lower back/buttocks, pain when urinating, urgent and increased frequency of urination, difficulty starting to urinate and painful ejaculations.

It is treated with medications such as antibiotics, painkillers and occasionally steroids. The condition usually resolves after a few weeks.

Joke: Doctor: "What brought you here today?"
Patient: "An ambulance!"

Chapter 13 - The Female Reproductive System

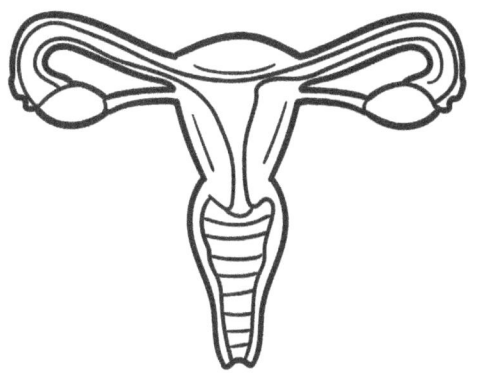

The Ovaries, Fallopian Tubes and Womb (medical term: Uterus).

The Female Reproductive System consists of the ovaries, fallopian tubes, womb, ovum cells and breasts.

The menstrual cycle is useful to understand before getting into this chapter. On Day 1 of a woman's period (first day of bleeding) an ovum cell is released from an ovary. The ovum lasts for just 24 hours and travels down the fallopian tube into the womb where it awaits a sperm cell to fertilise it.

If no sperm is present the lining of the womb (which has filled up with blood ready for fertilisation and implantation) sheds and the blood and ovum cells are released.

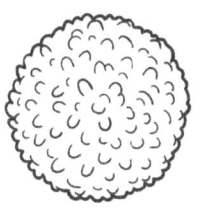

An Ovum

You'd be forgiven for thinking that this means there is only 24 hours a month when a female can get pregnant, but this is not the case.

This is because sperm can live inside a woman's body for 5-7 days, meaning that there is up to a 7 day window for conception every 28 days, providing that periods are regular.

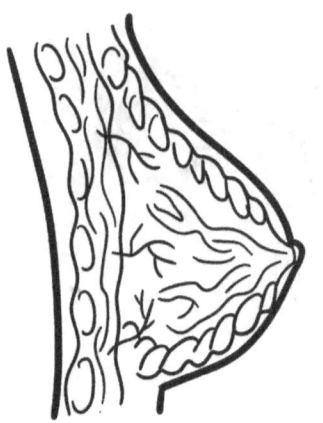

A Breast (side view)

The function of the breasts is to provide nutrition to a young infant up until 4-6 months of age when a baby is fully weaned onto solid foods. (This is despite what males of the species may *think* they are for.)

First Milk (medical term: Colostrum) is produced in the first 2-4 days and is full of good stuff, including compounds that support the immune, digestive and nutritional needs of the newborn.

Conception rates depend on so many factors, but most heterosexual couples will get pregnant within the first year of having sex without any form of contraception.

Joke: Gay/Lesbian couples may require help in the conception department. But gay/lesbian people are free to put in plenty of practice trying.

Conception problems can have a number of causes including:

❖ Eating disorders, obesity and excessive exercise as these all alter normal functioning of the menstrual system.

❖ Hormone imbalances, including conditions affecting the Thyroid (see p82-88), again as these can affect the normal functioning of the menstrual system.

❖ Infections of the reproductive system (in both females and males), usually sexually transmitted ones such as Chlamydia and Gonorrhea. Both are bacterial infections and treatable with antibiotics.

❖ Blocked fallopian tubes.

❖ Endometriosis (see below).

❖ Polycystic Ovary Syndrome (PCOS) (see below)

❖ Low sperm count in males (see p110).

❖ Being older in age 40+ years old in females. Fertility decreases in females with age.

❖ Menopause (depending on the stage and whether ovulation has stopped or not yet).

There are treatments to support people who have difficulties with conception, including lifestyle changes and In Vitro Fertilisation (IVF). The first step is for individuals to see their GP who will refer them to a Sexual & Reproductive Specialist.

Endometriosis is a condition in which cells/tissue grow outside of the womb (in places such as the ovaries & fallopian tubes) but acts like lining of the womb tissue - shedding each month. Symptoms of Endometriosis include:

❖ Lower abdominal pain - usually worse during a female's period.

❖ Debilitating period pain, that stops an individual from doing the activities of daily living.

❖ Pain during or after sex (female only).

❖ Pain urinating or opening bowels, nausea / vomiting on period.

❖ Constipation or loose stools during a period.

❖ Problems with getting pregnant due to decreased fertility.

There is no cure for Endometriosis, but there are treatments. Treatments include pain management medication, hormone medications (including oral contraceptive pills) and surgery to remove the affected tissue.

Fibroids are non-cancerous growths (I have no idea why they aren't called polyps) that grow in and around the womb. The exact cause(s) of Fibroids are unknown and some females with them may be unaware of them due to being asymptomatic (having no symptoms). Some women do have symptoms though and these can include abdominal pain, heavy/particularly painful periods, increased urination frequency, pain/discomfort during sex and constipation.

Fibroids treatment includes medications (including painkillers, hormones - usually oral contraceptive pills), insertion of a contraceptive Intrauterine System (IUS) - a plastic T shaped contraceptive method that contains progesterone and surgery.

Low sex drive (loss of libido) has the same causes as in males (see p107) and the same treatments - other than male specific treatments for Impotence.

Irregular and heavy periods are experienced by most women at some point in their lives. These usually either self-resolve or sometimes require lifestyle changes. Sometimes they can be treated with oral contraceptive pills. The Combined Pill contains both Oestrogen and Progesterone and puts the ovaries to sleep, having a break from taking the tablets 1 in every 3 weeks which provides an artificial bleed.

The Progesterone Only pill puts your ovaries to sleep and provides no bleed.

Both the Combined and Progesterone Only Pills take 7 days (one pill a day) to put the ovaries to sleep and it takes 7 days for the effects to wear off. If having sexual intercourse in the first 7 days of starting these pills it is recommended an alternative method of contraception is used (usually condoms) as the pills are not yet effective.

In the event of unprotected sex, the risk of pregnancy can be minimised by Emergency Contraception, this is a either an Intrauterine Device (IDU) (also known as the Copper Coil - interesting fact: copper is toxic to sperm cells) or a pill that can be taken within 120 hours of the sex. However the sooner Emergency Contraception, the lesser the risk of pregnancy.

Menopause is caused by a reduction in hormone levels and is a natural part of ageing in a female. Menopause symptoms vary from individual to individual but can include:

❖ Hot flushes, including shakes and sweats.

❖ Palpitations.

❖ Insomnia including night sweats and night terrors.

❖ Headaches / migraines.

❖ Changes to periods, including irregular periods and later periods stopping altogether.

❖ Changes to mood, including low mood, problems with concentrating (brain fog) and increased anxiety.

❖ Mouth / teeth sensitivity and problems.

❖ Recurrent urinary infections.

❖ Reduced sex drive and problems with vaginal dryness.

❖ Weight gain.

❖ Muscle aches and pains.

Treatments are those to manage symptoms and can include medications (such as hormone replacement therapy, antianxiety/antidepressants, painkillers, etc.), physio and occupational therapy.

Premature Ovarian Insufficiency (POI) is early on-set Menopause in a woman before the age of 40 years old. See Menopause above for further details of symptoms and treatments.

Ovarian Cysts are cysts that grow on either of the two ovaries. The cause is unknown. Cysts are fluid filled sacs. These often come and go on their own without any symptoms. But on occasion a cyst or cysts can cause pelvic pain and may need surgery to remove them if they grow too big.

Pelvic Prolapse or Pelvic Organ Prolapse is when the uterus, bladder, or top of the vagina move position and bulge into the lower vagina. It is caused by the pelvic floor muscles not being strong enough to support the organs and keep them in place. There is no immediate cure.

However there are treatments. Pelvic floor exercises can help, as can lifestyle changes such as losing weight. Medications may also be prescribed such as painkillers, anti-inflammatories and hormones. There are also a range of surgical treatment options that can resolve a pelvic prolapse.

Polycystic Ovary Syndrome (PCOS) is a condition that affects how the ovaries operate. To be diagnosed with PCOS you need to have at least two of the following:
1. Irregular periods.
2. Polycystic ovaries - ovaries that are enlarged due to follicles (fluid filled sacs that are not cysts - despite the name).
3. An increased amount of androgen hormones.

PCOS symptoms can include irregular/absent periods, difficulty getting pregnant, weight gain, excessive hair on face/back/chest/buttocks, acne and hair loss/hair thinning with no other cause (for other causes of hair loss see p31-33).

There is no cure for PCOS but there are treatments including lifestyle changes, medications (hormones including contraceptive oral pill, IUS insertion and medications for other symptoms), treatment for fertility issues and occasionally surgery.

Thrush (medical term: Candidosis) can occur in both females and males. In females it occurs in the vagina and sometimes the mouth. Thrush is caused by a fungal infection and is treated by antifungal topical cream and sometimes an oral tablet.

Vaginal Bacteriosis (VB) is a change to the bacteria in an individual's vagina and can have the following symptoms:

❖ A strong smelling discharge from the vagina, particularly after sex.

❖ A change in the consistency of vaginal discharge, for example it may become greyish and watery.

Treatment for VB is treated with medications including antibiotics. Although VB is not a sexually transmitted infection or disease (STI/STD), if an individual is sexually active their GP may recommend that they have a sexual health screen to rule out other causes of this vaginal discharge.

When a female is aroused the brain sends messages to the vagina to produce natural lubrication, Vaginal Dryness can affect any female and can have a number of causes including Menopause or not being sexually aroused at time of sexual intercourse or other sexual activity.

The easiest treatment for this is to use water-based lubricants, available at all Sexual Health Clinics.

A Note of Vaginal Dryness & Sex Workers

As Female Sex Workers are often not aroused at time of sexual intercourse or other sexual activity, they tend to be at higher risk of Vaginal Dryness. Sex Workers are recommended to use lubrication as required.

Sex Workers of both genders are also advised to always use condoms as they offer better protection against STIs/STDs, lubrication as required and have regular sexual health screening.

Chapter 14 - System Wide Malfunctions

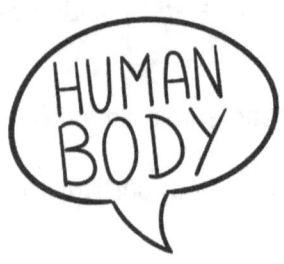

System Wide Malfunctions can affect any system in the body and usually affect more than one system.

Abscesses are the first malfunction, caused by a bacterial infection that can appear and grow anywhere. But most commonly occur in the teeth/gums, groin, around the anus, etc.

Treatment for abscesses include antibiotics, bursting the abscess to drain the pus and occasionally surgical drainage with a wound post op that needs packing.

Cancer can practically occur anywhere in the human body and is caused by a malfunction in the cell division process (medical term: Mitosis). Rather than creating two identical new cells, during the process a gene mutation occurs that creates a cancer cell. These then begin to reproduce causing cancer cells to spread. Cancer can affect practically any part of the body and vary in terms of their speed of duplication and spreading to other parts or systems of the body.

Symptoms of cancer depend on where the cancer is in the body. But general symptoms include:

❖ Extreme fatigue.

❖ A lump or swelling anywhere on the body.

❖ Pain/aches anywhere in the body.

❖ Weight Loss.

❖ New symptoms that don't appear to have any explanation.

❖ Night Sweats / A high temperature.

❖ Bleeding or bruising without good cause.

With cancer the earlier it is identified, the more treatment options there are and in most cases the better the outcomes. People can and do survive cancer, thanks to improved treatments.

Treatments for cancer include surgery to remove the cancerous cells, medicines, radiotherapy and chemotherapy. Successful cancer treatment depends on so many factors. There are many good books and websites that exist about the various forms of cancer. Please check these out for more specific information.

Chronic Fatigue Syndrome (medical term: Myalgic Encephalomyelitis or ME) is a chronic long term condition characterised by extreme fatigue and other symptoms. The cause of chronic fatigue syndrome is unknown and there is no cure for it.

In addition to extreme fatigue an individual with chronic fatigue syndrome will experience symptoms that include insomnia, cognition/memory problems, headaches, flu-like symptoms and elevated pulse rate with or without an irregular heart beat.

Treatments for chronic fatigue syndrome include CBT, energy management, medications and sometimes lifestyle changes.

Fibromyalgia is long term (3+ months) of pain throughout an individual's body, the exact cause of fibromyalgia is unknown. Other symptoms of fibromyalgia include extreme fatigue and issues with cognition/memory.

There is no cure for fibromyalgia. Treatments for fibromyalgia aim to improve quality of life and include exercise, talking therapies (such as general counselling & CBT) and medication.

Glandular Fever is a particularly nasty viral infection that usually affects adolescents and young adults. Symptoms include:
 ❖ A high temperature (over 37.5°C).

 ❖ Swollen glands.

 ❖ Sore throat.

- ❖ A rash.

- ❖ Headaches.

- ❖ Fatigue.

Glandular fever is treated by self-care at home and rarely needs medical input, unless the individual has other chronic conditions. Glandular fever is very infectious and is spread through spit, so sharing of knives/forks/spoons is not recommended.

Sepsis is a life threatening reaction to a bacterial infection, it used to be called blood poisoning. Symptoms include:
- ❖ **T**emperature - may be high or low.
- ❖ **I**nfection - there are signs/symptoms of an infection.
- ❖ **M**ental Decline - cognitive impairment/confusion is common in sepsis.
- ❖ **E**xteremy ill - the individual reports feeling extremely unwell.

Sepsis is a time sensitive condition and the Sepsis 6 should be completed **within 1 hour** of presentation:
1. Ensure senior doctor review.

2. Give oxygen if required.

3. Obtain intravenous access and take bloods (including blood cultures).

4. Give intravenous antibiotics (broad spectrum).

5. Give intravenous fluids.

6. Monitor all observations for any signs of further deterioration.

Chapter 15 - A Note on Trans & Non-Binary Issues

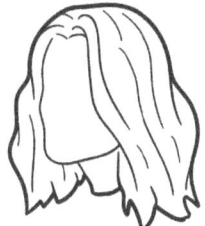

Those aware of Trans and Non-Binary issues will be aware that this book makes no reference to them.

There is a very good reason for this. I don't feel knowledgeable or skilled enough to write about these topics.

The best place I've found to get information is Sparkle - The National Transgender Charity, their website is: https://www.sparkle.org.uk/. They champion Trans inclusion and are a fabulous charity.

I would also like to remind all Healthcare Professionals of The Equality Act (2010) that legally protects individuals who are Trans or Non-Binary from discrimination when accessing services. Please remember that Trans and Non-Binary people regularly face stigma and discrimination in life without the need for it in healthcare services.

Trans and Non-Binary people are great educators, they will educate you about the issues they face if you ask respectfully and listen with genuine interest.

To my Trans and Non-Binary friends, there may be occasions when Healthcare Professionals may need to know what gender you were born. This is to diagnose, treat and minimise the risks of harm to you and others. For example, if having an x-ray. The Radiologist may need to know what gender you were born. This is to assess risk of pregnancy to prevent harm to an unborn child. This is just one example of many occasions when we may need this information.

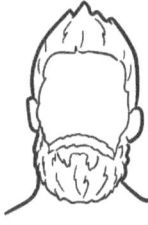

Please be understanding of this and don't be afraid to ask the reason why the Health Professional needs this information if unsure. They should be more than happy to answer.

Healthcare:
Clinical Excellence

Appendix A - Clinical Assessment

A good clinical assessment leads to excellent patient care. Always start where possible by introducing yourself and explaining your role. Always ask the patient what has brought them to see you today. Sometimes patients or their relatives are able to give you lots of valuable information. These are the questions I ask every patient that I see:

> ➢ What has brought you to see me today?
> ➢ What are you concerned about?
> ➢ How long have you felt this way/had these concerns?
> ➢ Do you have any medical conditions that I need to know about?
> ➢ Do you take any medication and what have you taken today?
> ➢ Are you allergic to anything?
> ➢ Is there anything else that I need to know?

After these initial questions, a clinical assessment should be undertaken using the A, B, C, D, E approach:

1. Airway -
Is the patient able to maintain their own airway without support or assistance?

Consider:

❖ The patient's position on the bed/trolly - a slight adjustment in positioning may enable them to open their airway more easily.

❖ Are there any unusual noises such as Wheezes, Grunting, Coughing, Gurgling or a Stridor? These are indications that the patient is struggling with maintaining their airway or breathing problems.

❖ Is the patient grabbing at their throat or do they appear panicked? This might be because they aren't able to breathe properly. It is completely normal for a patient to panic if they feel that they can't inhale enough air or are short of breath.

❖ Check the patient's chest and abdomen for a see-sawing movement. This can be an indication of injury through trauma, inhibition of gas exchange in the lungs or respiratory fatigue. These patients are at high risk of requiring ventilation. You should be really concerned if you see this and seek immediate review by a Doctor.

❖ Is there a visible blockage in the throat? A strong back slap or the Heimlich Maneuver (in adults only) may be successful in removal of the obstruction.

In the cases of babies and children: if you can see an object in their month, try to remove it with your fingers or forceps.

For babies, turn them over so that their face is pointing towards the floor (gravity also helps in this case) and x5 back slaps followed by rubbing and vigorous circular rubbing in the centre of the back. This may dislodge a blockage. However throat and mouth blockages in babies should be extremely rare as they take a liquid diet and are not yet mobile enough to get and put small objects in their mouth. In these cases after the baby is stabilised questions should be asked as to how this occurred.

For older children encourage them to cough (especially if they are already doing so) and if required deliver back slaps with them leaning forward.

As with all clinical activities, only do what you have been trained to do and feel competent to do. If you're unsure or don't feel competent, get immediate help from colleagues.

❖ Does the patient require oxygen delivered through a high concentration mask?

❖ If the airway is compromised by mucus or other similar substance? Consider the use of suction to remove the substance.

2. **Breathing** -
   Observe Respiratory Rate (breaths per minute), these days we often have technology that will monitor respiratory rate. But you can't beat looking at your patient, rather than a screen. Looking at your patient will give you much more information than looking at a screen.

   Observe oxygen saturation levels.

Consider:

❖ Depth of breathing? Use of accessory muscles? Both of these give you an indication of how hard they are working to breathe. The deeper the breath and the greater use of the accessory muscles the more respiratory distress the patient is in.

❖ Does the child patient display a recession or a tracheal tug? In children these are signs of significant respiratory distress.

❖ Unusual breathing sounds such as grunting, auditable wheeze, can give a good indication of breathing difficulties and the urgency for immediate treatment.

❖ Nasal flaring can be a sign of respiratory distress.

❖ Marked use of the diaphragm indicates difficulty breathing.

❖ Colour of the patient can be an indicator of breathing problems. If they are pale or grey looking, it shows that they are not getting enough oxygen.

❖ Ask if the patient has any pre-existing breathing conditions such as Asthma or COPD.

3. Circulation -

Take the patient's pulse rate and blood pressure (BP). Again a manual pulse rate taken on the patient's wrist (peripheral pulse) or neck (central pulse) will give you much more information than looking at a monitor's screen.

Do a peripheral and central capillary refill time.

Take the patient's temperature.

Consider:

❖ A strong and bounding pulse indicates that the cardiovascular system is working hard.

❖ A weak and thready peripheral pulse or absence of a peripheral pulse indicates that the patient is going into shock or is already in it. Shock is pre-terminal and can lead to death if not immediately treated. Escalate a weak and thready peripheral pulse or absence of a peripheral pulse to a Doctor and assertively request an immediate assessment from them.

- ❖ A reduced level of consciousness, a patient being confused, a patient being sleepy or asleep are all signs of circulatory system problems. If the patient is drowsy, talk to them to try and maintain consciousness. If the patient is asleep try to wake them. If they are unresponsive, press the emergency buzzer for immediate help.
- ❖ When assessing level of consciousness be aware of things that can affect a patient's level of consciousness such as alcohol or having taken an overdose of sedative medications.
- ❖ Get Intravenous (IV) access as soon as possible and take standard bloods. Sometimes blood cultures may also be required.
- ❖ Monitoring of urinary output may be required to ensure a careful fluid balance in the body. Sometimes when close monitoring is required a catheter may need to be inserted.
- ❖ Intravenous fluids may be prescribed and need to be administered.
- ❖ In some circumstances blood transfusions may be required. Blood transfusions may be full or part of blood products (such as just red blood cells or platelets). It will depend on the cause of blood loss or which conditions they have and how they affect the cardiovascular system.
- ❖ Complete a blood sugar (BM) test. Sometimes a late sign of a low or very high blood sugar can be a reduced level of consciousness or unresponsiveness.
- ❖ On rare occasions, when the circulatory system is in shutdown, gaining IV access may be impossible. In these cases Intraosseous Access (IA) may be sought. IA is usually obtained by a senior Doctor skilled to do so.
- ❖ A low BP is a sign of hypovolemic shock.
- ❖ A high BP can be caused by stress, pain or can be pre-existing. Always ask if they have a history of high BP, if they take any medications for this and if they have taken their medication today?

❖ A high temperature (more than 37.5°C) can indicate an infection. Infections can be either caused by bacteria or viruses. Bacterial infections are usually treated with either intravenous or oral antibiotics. Viral infections are usually left for the body's immune system to resolve. Very occasionally in life threatening situations, such as in Intensive Care Units (ICUs) antiviral medications may be used.

❖ A low temperature (less than 36°C) may be treated by wrapping the patient in extra blankets and sometimes with use of a bear hugger as well (a plastic blanket with a machine that pumps hot air inside of the blanket).

❖ Ask the patient: Have you ever been diagnosed with any blood borne viruses? Are you on any medications for these and if so, have you taken the medication today?

4. Disability -

Assess consciousness level: Alert, Verbal, Pain, Unresponsive (AVPU). The Glasgow Coma Scale (GCS) can also be useful to assess consciousness level and is commonly used in cases of head injuries.

If not already done, complete a blood sugar test. In the result of a high blood sugar (above 13 mmol/l), a ketone test should be completed.

Assess pupil sizes and reaction to light times - monitor this on a regular basis.

Observe for and appropriately treat seizures.

Assess pain and respond appropriately.

Consider:
❖ What could be the underlying cause of a reduced level of consciousness? What treatment does the patient need for the underlying cause?

❖ Ensure that the patient's level of consciousness is regularly reassessed to identify any deterioration early.

- Treat low blood sugars (below 4 mmol/l) with oral fast acting sugary food, followed by some food containing slower acting carbohydrates. Sometimes IV glucose may be given, particularly if the patient is unconscious.
- Treat high blood sugars (more than over 11 mmol/l) following local policies and procedures. This might include a stat dose of subcutaneous insulin and in more severe cases intravenous insulin on a sliding scale.
- Any pupils particularly pin pricked (small) or large should be escalated and continued to be monitored on a regular basis.
- Pupils that are slow and sluggish to respond to light can indicate intracranial swelling (swelling of the brain). A CT scan of the head may be undertaken to diagnose intracranial swelling/rising intracranial pressure. Intracranial swelling/pressure can result in death.

It can be treated by tilting the bed 30° so that the head is an upright position at all times to help with cerebral drainage, sometimes with a medicine called Mannitol and in rare cases surgery to fracture the skull to allow the brain to swell safely without crushing the brain stem (a crushed brain stem always results in death).

5. Exposure -
Examine the patient from head to toe, front and back. What you're looking for is any deformities (swelling, lumps, any shortening and rotation of one leg, a bone sticking out of the skin, etc.). These other injuries may need to be treated.

Consider:
- Where on the body the abnormality is and what this could mean for what is going on inside the patient's body.
- Document your findings on a body map in the patient's records and escalate as appropriate.

Repeat the A, B, C, D, E assessment process as required and always remember to document the assessment, plan of care and treatments given.

Appendix B - All Age Observational Norms

Here are rough observational norms for all ages (from birth to adulthood).

Please note: That these might vary slightly from those listed on your local observation charts and Early Warning Score (EWS) systems.

Respiratory Rate

Age	Respirations (Per Minute)
Newborn	30-60
6 Months	30-45
1-2 Years	25-35
3-6 Years	20-30
7+ Years	20-25
Adults	12-18

Pulse Rate

Age	Pulse (Beats Per Minute)
Newborn	100-180
Less Than 3 Months Old	100-220
3 Months-2 Years Old	80-150
3-10 Years	60-100
11+ Years	60-100
Adults	60-100

Blood Pressure

Age	Systolic	Diastolic
Infant (6 Months)	75-105	40-70
Toddler (2 Years)	75-110	45-80
School Age (7 Years)	75-115	45-80
Adolescent (15 Years)	100-145	60-95
Adult	Less than 140	Less than 90

Temperature
A normal temperature range for all ages is 36°C – 37.5°C.

Oxygen Saturations (O2 Sats)
A normal O2 sats range for all ages is 95%-100%. In patients with COPD, the normal range is 88%-92% due the condition.

Patients with low O2 sats may have a bluish tinge to their fingernails, lips and occasionally skin. Patients displaying any sort of bluish tinge should be immediately reviewed by a doctor.

Blood Sugar (BM)
A normal blood sugar for a non-diabetic for all ages is 4-8 mmol/l.

For diabetics an acceptable range is 5-9 mmol/l.

If blood sugars are over 17 mmol/l or repeatedly over 13 mmol/l (medical term: Hyperglycemia), a ketone test should be completed and results (which are instant) should be immediately responded to, this prevents ketoacidosis (see more about diabetes on p48-59).

If blood sugars are below 4 mmol/l (medical term: Hypoglycemia). The patient should be given some fast acting sugar, followed by some slower acting carbohydrates.

Documentation
All observations should be documented, along with any responses to high or low readings.

Influences on Observational Norms
There are a number of things that can influence observational norms, including:

❖ Pain - This can increase all observational norms, with the exception of temperature.

❖ Infections - This can increase all observational norms, including temperature.

❖ Internal/External Bleeding - This can increase/decrease observations depending on how much blood is lost out of the cardiovascular system.

   Please note: That a decreasing blood pressure is a pre-terminal sign and warrants immediate medical review.

❖ Recent Exercise - This can increase most observations (Respiratory Rate, Pulse, Blood Pressure), but can occasionally lower BM.

   Example from Practice: If a patient has just been for a cigarette, wait 10 minutes before taking and recording observations due to the impact of the walk outside and of Nicotine (see below).

❖ Dietary Intake - Will increase BM in diabetics, particularly if food contains sugars or carbohydrates.

❖ Body Size - A larger person is likely to have higher than normal observations, whereas a smaller person may have slightly lower observational norms than average.

❖ Exercise Routines - Regular exercise lowers Respiratory Rate, Pulse & Blood Pressure.

Example from Practice: I once took the Pulse rate of a 18 year old male who had a Pulse rate of 40 BPM. He was sat up talking with me. He confirmed that he regularly exercises 4-5 times a week, for an hour each time.

❖ Medications - A wide range of medications can increase or decrease observational norms. There are too many to list here.

Example from Practice: Salbutamol, administered via inhaler or nebuliser to improve breathing causes the heart rate to increase.

Another Example from Practice: Medications used to manage ADHD are stimulants (see below) and can increase Pulse Rate and Blood Pressure.

❖ Conditions / Diseases - A wide range of conditions can increase or decrease observational norms. There are too many to list here, but hopefully through reading this book you have been made aware of many of them.

❖ Stimulant Substance Use - Stimulant substances include:
Nicotine/Smoking
Caffeine
Cocaine
Ecstasy/MDMA
Amphetamines
Crystal Methamphetamine

Please consider the effects of poly substance use! Using multiple drugs that are stimulants/depressants/hallucinogens.

Be aware that the patient might think they have taken one drug, when in fact they have taken another.

❖ Depressant Substance Use

Alcohol
Benzodiazepines
Heroin
Methadone (including Street Bought)
GHB/GBL
Ketamine
Glues, Gasses & Aerosols (Volatile Substance Abuse)

Please consider the effects of poly substance use! Using multiple drugs that are stimulants/depressants/hallucinogens.

Be aware that the patient might think they have taken one drug, when in fact they have taken another.

❖ Hallucinogenic Substance Use
Cannabis
LSD
Magic Mushrooms
Spice (New Psychoactive Substance)

Please consider the effects of poly substance use! Using multiple drugs that are stimulants/depressants/hallucinogens.

Be aware that the patient might think they have taken one drug, when in fact they have taken another.

❖ Mental / Emotional State - Being confused, anxious, having a panic attack or being stressed can cause increases in observational norms.

❖ Environmental Exposure (Chemicals/Poisons) - Chemicals or poisons can cause altered observational norms. Use a poisons database for treatment algorithms.

❖ Environmental Exposure (Temperatures) - Exposure to high or low temperatures can lead to increased or decreased observational norms. The most effective treatment in these cases is to treat accordingly.

If the patient is too hot, reduce the amount of clothing, provide cold drinks (to lower core temperature) and care for in a cool environment.

If the patient is too cold, give additional blankets, use a bear hugger and care for in a warmer environment.

Appendix C - The Nursing Model of Care

The Nursing Model of Care, diagram below has been around for as long as I can remember. I unfortunately couldn't find a reference online to give credit to its makers.

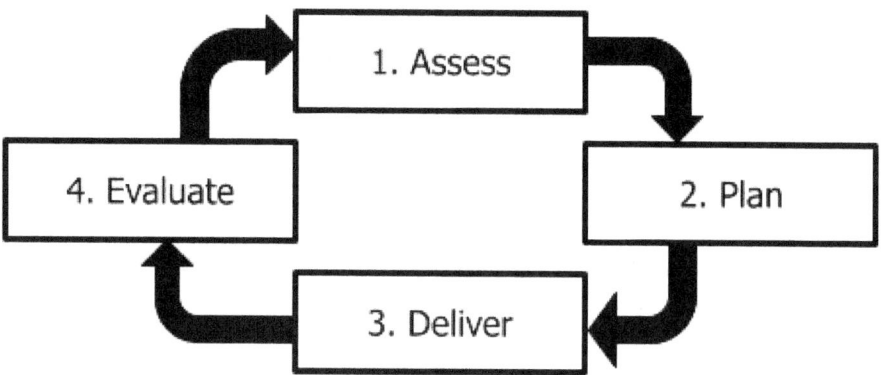

Since this original model, many others have developed their own models of care, but all essentially based on the foundations of this framework.

1. Assess

In an emergency assessment, use the A, B, C, D, E approach as outlined in Appendix A and take observations comparing them to norms, see Appendix B.

Assessments where an emergency isn't present should be both comprehensive and holistic. To undertake this sort of assessment you will need to build a good and trusting rapport with the patient and possibly relatives as well.

A comprehensive and holistic assessment should cover:
* ❖ Presenting issue, including current symptoms and past/current treatments along with any outcomes.

* ❖ Patients' presentation on assessment, details of any relatives present, documentation of informed consent and that the patient understands confidentiality, its limits and how their data will be used.

- ❖ GP details.

- ❖ Patient's goal: What do they want to get out of your intervention today?

- ❖ Past medical history including any diagnoses or symptoms of physical & mental illnesses, along with current treatments.

- ❖ Current medications, compliance and allergy details.

- ❖ Details of activities of daily living.

- ❖ Details of lifestyle: Smoking status, alcohol consumption details and substances used.

- ❖ In some cases a Mental Capacity Assessment or other cognitive assessment.

- ❖ Details of any Deprivation of Liberty Safeguards (DoLS) in place and their rationale.

- ❖ Next of kin details, support networks, any caring responsibilities they may have and any support they currently get (e.g. from Social Workers/Carers/etc.).

- ❖ An agreement of what information can be shared with whom and under what circumstances between the patient and your organisation.

- ❖ Identification of services involved and reasons.

- ❖ Employment or benefit details, details of any financial concerns.

- ❖ Armed forces & veteran status.

- ❖ Identification of autism or learning disability needs.

❖ The identification of any safeguarding issues (both for adults and children).

❖ Details of any on-going and relevant Police investigations or warrants out for their arrest.

❖ Any specific assessment tools relating to your specific field of practice such as pain assessment tools, the Bristol Stool Chart, the Patient Health Questionnaire, GAD (Generalised Anxiety Disorder) Assessment, SADQ (Severity of Alcohol Dependence Questionnaire).

❖ A list of immediate actions including any referrals to other internal departments or external services, as agreed with the patient.

2. Plan
A care plan is a list of identified health needs (identified from the assessment), treatment actions, who is responsible for completing the actions, expected outcomes and dates to review individual actions and overall care plan.

To ensure clinical excellence all care plans should be written in a way that is SMART (Specific, Measurable, Achievable, Realistic/Resourced & Timescaled).

Many Nurses complete a care plan, file it away in the patient notes and never look at it again. Some organisations now have standardised care plans on their Electronic Patient Records (EPRs) system for particular diseases/conditions.

Best clinical practice is to update the care plan as things change for the patient. This means that realistically the plan of care should be updated a minimum of once a day.

Nurses tend to "do" to patients, rather than do "with" patients. This is often due to trying to be efficient and save time. But when creating or updating a care plan, it is crucial that it should be done in collaboration with patients (and relatives where appropriate).

3. Deliver

Delivery of patient care may include a wide range of activities including: support with activities of daily living (such as ensuring adequate intake of diet and fluids, washing/bathing, etc.), prescribing/administration of medicines, referrals to and liaison with other professionals/specialities, taking observations, taking blood samples, liaising with relatives, etc.

All care and treatments should be delivered using a non-judgemental approach, being sensitive to cultural needs/wishes and with compassion and empathy.

All care and treatments should be completed with the informed consent of the patient (from 16 years old and older). There may be cases where gaining informed consent is not possible, for example due to the patient being unconscious or having a cognitive impairment. In these cases healthcare professionals should act in the best interests of the patient.

In the case of children (under 13 years old) informed consent should be sought from parents/carers with legal responsibility for the child.

In the case of young people (aged 13-15 years old) a Fraser Assessment should be undertaken to see if they have capacity to consent to treatment. A Fraser Assessment considers:
1. The age, maturity and mental capacity of the young person.

2. The individual's understanding of the advantages, disadvantages and long term consequences of having care/treatment.

3. The risks and implications of giving informed consent or withholding it. Bearing in mind that the healthcare professional has a duty to ensure that the young person's best interests are met.

4. How well the young person can demonstrate true understanding of the information explained to them.

5. Their ability to explain the rationale for giving or withholding consent taking into account all the above.

6. That a discussion has taken place with the young person about whether they want to inform their parents/carers and their reasons for how they feel about this.

7. That the care/treatment is not a safeguarding issue. Safeguarding issues override confidentiality and the need for consent for care/treatment.

Most settings have a form for Assessing Fraser Competence, as well as good safeguarding children policies/procedures. If you are ever unsure, seek advice and support from someone more senior or a Safeguarding Specialist.

Care/treatment should be delivered confidentially, unless the patient or someone else is at risk of harm.

Care/treatment should be inline with best available evidence-based practice and guidelines - such as National Institute for Clinical Excellence (NICE) guidelines. This includes infection prevention measures such as hand washing and Aseptic Non Touch Technique (where appropriate).

Care/treatment is more than just treating what condition the patient has come to you with, it is also about the prevention of further harm. Further harm prevention could involve rotating the patient to prevent pressure sores, actions to minimise the risk of falls, etc.

Care/treatment may include public health work such as educating the patient and their relatives on their diseases, treatments and how to stay well in the longer term. You should be able to answer any questions asked, but if you are not able to, always seek advice from colleagues (including Specialists) rather than giving out vague or incorrect information.

All care/treatment should be fully documented (see Documentation Appendix on p154-157 for more information).

4. Evaluate

Evaluation of care should be undertaken whenever something changes, following an intervention or at regular intervals during care/treatment.

The exact frequency of evaluating care will depend on your service, for example Wards in Hospitals might evaluate care either once a shift or once a day. But in the community these might be less regular, say once every 4-6 weeks, as they may only see a patient for an hour per week.

Once care has been evaluated, the patient should be re-assessed for any outstanding or additional needs that have developed and the cycle as indicated in the model above should be repeated. This is until care/treatments are completed or the patient is discharged from your care.

Failure to evaluate care has been identified in a number of Serious Case Reviews and Coroner Inquests where patient's have deteriorated due to an underlying/concurrent conditions or in the cases of misdiagnosis.

Appendix D - Communication is Key

Communication with patients, relatives and colleagues of all disciplines is key to safe and effective care. Here are some tips that if followed will improve your communication skills:

1. Introduce yourself, explain your role/task, allow time for questions and reassure patients. Always show empathy.

2. Ask open questions. These allow people to explain vital contextual information.

3. Take the time to summarise what has been said, to check that you have fully understood someone.

4. If in doubt about what someone has said, ask them to repeat it. If you don't understand what someone has said, ask them to explain it in another way or explain their thinking/rationale.

5. If you're receiving complex information, write it down in chronological order. Use bullet points if necessary.

6. When it comes to patient safety or trying to highlight deterioration in a patient, don't be afraid to be assertive and back up your concerns with evidence (e.g. an up-to-date set of observations).

7. Sometimes there are barriers to effective communication such as a language barrier, a patient being non-verbal or a patient being hard of hearing.

   In the case of a language barrier, arrange for an interpreter, never use family members.

   In the case of a patient being non-verbal listen closely to carers who will explain behavioural cues and observe body language closely.

   In the case of a patient being hard of hearing, writing information down on paper or providing written literature may help.

8. Establish a rapport with all those you communicate with. This can be done by active listening, paying attention to what they are saying and being honest at all times.

9. When expressing your concerns about a patient to a colleague (of any discipline) start with the most important concern first.

10. Keep patients informed. Let them know what they are waiting for, what is likely to happen next and estimated timescales.

11. Explain Ward/Department routines to patients and provide contact details for relatives/carers to keep in touch.

12. Allow time for patients to ask any questions they have and answer them as fully as possible.

13. If a patient is defensive or aggressive, there is usually a good reason for this. Try to establish the root cause of this behaviour and address it.

14. Remember what may be important to you, might not be as important to the patient, relatives or other professionals. Ask them what's important to them, what their goals are and negotiate to see if there is some compromise where both parties can achieve their goals.

15. Document all communications effectively and accurately. Do this as soon as possible after the event, while the details are fresh in your mind.

16. Be aware of different cultural backgrounds than your own. This will help you navigate culturally sensitive conversations and care.

17. Be positive and always try to remain calm. Smile and use manners. Patients, relatives and other professionals will pick up any anxiety or worry that you express and focus on it.

18. Be aware of your own body language and make sure it conveys what you are trying to express verbally.

19. Adapt your communication style to different patient groups. For example, if speaking with a child, get down to their level to make eye contact. This is less intimidating than towering over a child.

20. Be aware of pronouns, if in doubt ask the patient which they prefer and use them.

21. Never assume anything, if in doubt ask.

22. Give praise and encouragement as appropriate.

23. Suggest distraction activities as appropriate.

24. Use humour, but only in appropriate situations. If you are unsure whether a situation is appropriate to use humour, it probably isn't. In these circumstances, don't make jokes or use humour.

Appendix E - Situation, Background, Assessment & Recommendations (SBAR) Handovers

The SBAR was developed for use in nuclear submarines. The aviation industry adopted it, followed by healthcare systems across the world. The SBAR handover system is recommended by NHS England.

There are many benefits to an SBAR handover including:

❖ Improved and structured communication - Between all healthcare professionals.

❖ Improved patient safety - A reduced risk of errors or care/treatments being missed.

❖ Improved efficiency - Handovers are shorter and focus on the essential information.

❖ It is a versatile model - It can be used verbally and in documentation (ideally both in handover).

❖ It is a well known model by most healthcare professionals, is easy to remember and learn.

This is what each section of SBAR should include:

Situation

1. The patient's details should be included in Situation. This should include full name, date of birth and any identification numbers (such as hospital number/NHS Number/Community Caseload Number).

2. Your details including: full name, role, location) and contact details (telephone number and/or email address).

3. Patient current observations. Your concerns about the patient.

Background

1. Reason for Patient's admission/attendance at clinic.

2. Medical history including current diseases/conditions and past surgical procedures.

3. Working diagnosis or symptoms.

4. Allergies and current medications.

5. Normal mobility (i.e. mobile & independent) and cognitive functioning. Current mobility and details of any cognitive impairment.

Assessment
1. Current patient observations outside of norms and what care/treatment has been given to stabilise these.

   Remember: You should never move a patient who isn't clinically stable to another Ward/Department and never discharge them home.

2. What tests/investigations the patient has had and any results / when results are likely to be available.

3. Details of any treatment pathways/algorithms the patient is on.

Recommendations
1. List care/treatments outstanding. This could include repeat tests/investigations, medications, referrals on to specialists and for surgical procedures. If there is a timescale for these, make sure to make this clear.

2. Always recommend observation frequency, doctor/surgeon review, specialist assessment and to administer medications as prescribed.

3. Detail any care plans and when they are due for review.

4. Detail any communication plan to update next of kin or relatives, in the case that the patient is not able to do this for themselves.

It is good practice to have both a verbal and written documented handover. If in receipt of handover:

❖ Don't be afraid to make notes of actions that need completing and timescales.

❖ Check anything you don't understand the rationale for.

❖ Summarise the handover and in particular the recommendations back to the professional giving the handover. This ensures correct understanding.

Joke: There's new research showing that diarrhoea is hereditary. Apparently, it runs in your jeans.

Appendix F - The Specialists

There are Specialists Doctors, Nurses, Physiotherapists, Occupational Therapists, Radiologists, Pharmacists, Social Workers, Counsellors, Psychologists, Gynecologists, Midwives, Play Specialists, Youth Workers and a whole array of other professionals within the healthcare system. Some Specialities include:

- ❖ Acute Medicine
- ❖ Aesthetics
- ❖ Alcohol & Substance Use
- ❖ Allergy & Immunology
- ❖ Cardiology
- ❖ Children & Young People
- ❖ Dermatology
- ❖ Ear, Nose & Throat
- ❖ Emergency Care
- ❖ Endocrinology & Diabetes
- ❖ Gastroenterology
- ❖ General Practice
- ❖ Genetics
- ❖ Geriatric Medicine
- ❖ Gynecology & Obstetrics
- ❖ Health Visiting
- ❖ Intensive Care
- ❖ Learning Disability & Autism
- ❖ Mental Health, both Adult & Child
- ❖ Neurosurgery / Neuroscience
- ❖ Occupational Health
- ❖ Oncology (cancer screening, diagnosis and treatment)
- ❖ Ophthalmology
- ❖ Palliative / End of Life
- ❖ Pathology
- ❖ Plastics
- ❖ Public Health
- ❖ Respiratory
- ❖ School Nursing
- ❖ Sexual & Reproductive Health
- ❖ Trauma & Orthopedics
- ❖ Urology
- ❖ Vascular Surgery

Specialist professionals have the following role:

1. To assess and plan care for complex patients.

2. To undertake complex clinical procedures and treatments.

3. To provide advice, information and support for how you care for patients.

4. To develop policies, procedures and strategies to guide how you care for patients.

5. To provide training around their speciality.

6. To undertake clinical audits and other quality improvement programmes to improve clinical practice.

7. To contribute to research and developing evidence-based practice. Activities include supporting the development of NICE Guidelines and publishing research papers.

It would always be advisable for you to follow the advice and information of Specialists. However if you are ever unsure of the advice given, ask the Specialist to explain their rationale and if you are still unsure you should escalate your concerns to your line manager.

Joke: What's the difference between a GP and a Specialist?
One treats what you have, the other thinks you have what he treats.

Appendix G - Medication Tips for Healthcare Professionals

When prescribing or administering medication healthcare professionals should ensure:

1. Prescribing for / administering to the right patient. Check full name, date of birth and number identifiers.

2. Check the British National Formulary (BNF) or equivalent for appropriate dosages and contraindications or cautions.

3. You are aware of any allergies the patient has and conditions that might be contraindications.

4. Prescribe / Administer the right drug, at the right dose, at the right time and by the right route.

5. Be aware of the possible side effects of any medication given and when necessary prescribe / administer other medications to treat side effects.

6. When administering medications observe for an adverse reaction, such as anaphylaxis. If administering intravenous (IV) medications and you observe a reaction, stop administration immediately. Call for help and use an anaphylaxis kit, as you will have been trained to do so.

7. Document medication prescribed / administered on Drugs Cardex or electronic medication system.

On occasion you may be required to convert units, if you are required to do so, use this formula:

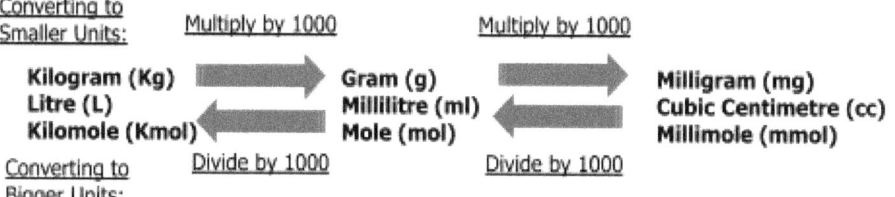

When calculating medications for children and adolescents, you should use this formula:

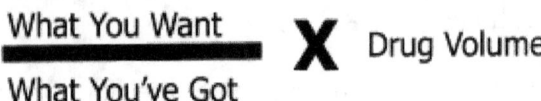

$$\frac{\text{What You Want}}{\text{What You've Got}} \quad \textbf{X} \quad \text{Drug Volume}$$

Joke: What's the difference between an oral and a rectal thermometer?
The taste.

Appendix H - Dealing with an Error

Unfortunately from time to time errors occur in healthcare. These errors can include (but are by no means limited to):

❖ Medication Errors - Prescribing/Administration of the wrong medication to the wrong patient, giving the wrong dose or by the wrong route, etc.

❖ Infection Prevention Measures Failures - Not washing hands leading to the spread of infections, not using Antiseptic Non Touch Technique.

❖ Pressure Sores - Caused by not rotating an immobile patient often enough.

❖ Deterioration in Physical/Mental Health - Caused by poor monitoring or timely assessment/input by specialists.

❖ Falls - Cause by poor monitoring of patients at risk of falls or by environmental factors such as wet floors.

❖ Wrong Surgical Procedures/procedures done on the wrong part of the body - Caused by lack of safety measures and use of safety checklists.

❖ Failure in Tests/Investigations - Caused by poor communication, lack of clinical skills or knowledge.

❖ Equipment Failures - Caused by not maintaining machines or inappropriately trained staff.

❖ Omissions - Caused by professionals not speaking up when something hasn't been completed or when they can foresee problems/issues with care.

Prevention of errors is better than allowing errors to occur. We prevent errors in healthcare by Risk Assessment & Risk Management Plans, ensuring patients are regularly reviewed, spotting potential errors and taking steps to avoid them occurring (such as the use of red name bands in patients with allergies) and good handovers.

However sometimes errors can and do occur, despite prevention measures. In the case of an error take the following steps:

1. Ensure Patient Safety - Get the patient reviewed by Doctors, prescribe/administer any reversal drugs (such as Naloxone), monitor closely.

2. Inform your Line Manager - Or Professional In Charge of the shift.

3. Review Care Plans, Risk Assessments & Risk Management Plans.

4. Inform the Patient and their Relatives (with informed consent) of the error sensitivity and of immediate actions taken.

5. Document your Actions taken.

6. Complete an Incident Report - So that lessons can be learned to prevent future occurrences of the same or similar errors.

7. Attend/Complete any training to skill you up in preventing errors, such as moving and handling training, anaphylaxis, falls prevention, medicines management, etc.

8. In some cases - Complete a Root Cause Analysis (RCA) to identify the root causes of the error and to recommend actions to prevent it occuring again.

Throughout the process of dealing with an error, remain calm, keep patient safety as the focus and be honest about any mistakes that you may have made.

Appendix I - Documentation Tips for Healthcare Professionals

If you don't document it, then it didn't happen. How many times have we heard this as healthcare professionals? Too often, but from a legal perspective it's true. Here are some documentation tips:

1. If your notes are written make sure they are legible. Illegible notes don't stand up in a coroner's inquest or court of law.

2. Make sure your notes are dated, timed, signed, name, role, location and NMC/GMC Registration Pin/Number. You can get stamps now that serve to clearly give your full name, role and NMC/GMC Registration Pin/Number.

3. Write up your notes as soon after activity as possible. Include relevant details. Relevant details include:

❖ Reason for contact/intervention.

❖ Details of any tests/investigations undertaken and results.

❖ Patient's concerns/comments and how you responded to these.

❖ Relatives concerns/comments and how you responded to this.

❖ Details of the patient's physical, mental and emotional state. It is good practice to include evidence to support these statements. For example:
Patient appeared agitated as evident by him pacing back and forth in the bay and clenching and unclenching his fists.

❖ Referrals on to Specialities and reasons for this. Details of whom you spoke with when you made the referral, including full name, job title and phone number.

❖ Liaison with other professionals or relatives. Details of whom you spoke with, including full name, job title/relationship to the patient and phone number.

❖ Details of any disclosures - including being victim of domestic abuse, rape/sexual assault, victim of crime, etc. and what you did about it, including exactly what was said to the patient and actions completed to safeguard the patient.

❖ Any offer of a chaperone and the patient's response.

❖ Care/Treatment updates, for example:
Received a call from John Smith (Lab Technician) who advised to change antibiotics to Co-Amoxiclav due to bacteria not being responsive to current antibiotics. Informed Dr Khan (FY1 Doctor) who updated the prescription. Antibiotics given as prescribed and as Drug Kardex indicates.

❖ Details of any meetings (such as MDT Meetings, Strategy Meetings or Core Group Meetings), including who was there, details of the discussions and agreed actions/outcomes.

❖ Details of any observed deterioration in patients, details of whom you have escalated it to and any response to your escalation.

4. Documentation should be objective and include facts. Don't include opinions, guesses or judgmental comments.

5. Abbreviations and acronyms should be avoided at all costs. Some healthcare organisations have approved lists of acronyms that can be used in notes. But if in doubt initially write it out in full, e.g. Blood Pressure (BP). Further occurrences can then be used as BP, as you have previously explained what this means by writing it out in full.

6. Don't use vague terms like 'on-going management.' As these terms mean nothing.

7. You can reference other documentation. For example, for further details see Care Plan dated.

8. Do include a plan of what will happen next.

9. Do document any use of preventative measures to keep a patient safe. This includes use of call bells, bed rails, 1-2-1 patient observation, etc.

10. If documenting care/treatment after the event. Start the entry with 'Written in retrospect' and include a reason as to why this documentation was delayed.

11. Never document care/treatments in advance, as the care/treatments might not be able to be delivered at the time you intend or may not happen the way you think they will.

12. When dealing with sensitive matters, it is useful to have another colleague present. Always detail the full name, job title and role of the colleague present.

13. Remember that management, the patient themselves or their relatives may request to see their notes through Medical Records. So never write anything that could be viewed as unsubstantiated or judgemental.

14. Any errors should also be documented with full details of how the error occurred and what you did about it.

15. Delays in care/treatments should be documented along with reasons for these delays, whom you've escalated it to and their responses.

16. You can include your rationale for your actions. You can also reference local policies/procedures and nationally agreed guidelines (such as NICE Guidelines). For example:

Patient doesn't appear to be oriented to place and date. I asked the patient where he is and he said 'at home.' I asked him if he knew the date, he said he did not. As the patient has previously been oriented to place and date, escalated to Dr Khan (FY1 Doctor) and made Sarah Davies (Charge Nurse) aware in line with Trust's Escalation Policy.
Plan:
1) Set of physical Observations to check for deterioration.

2) *BM as patient is diabetic.*
3) *Review recent blood tests results to check for possible causes of lack of orientation.*
4) *Medical Review by Dr Khan and then update plan of care as indicated.*

Joke: What are the ABC's of emergency medicine for Junior Doctors?
Assess from the doorway.
Back away slowly.
CT scan.

Appendix J - Useful Resources

Here are some useful resources and organisations:

Action Cerebral Palsy - Is a charity that aims to campaign for and provide information to the public about cerebral palsy.
Website: https://actioncp.org/

Action On Pain - Provides advice and information for people affected by chronic pain.
Website: https://action-on-pain.co.uk/

Age UK - A charity that provides information, advice and support for older people.
Website: https://www.ageuk.org.uk/

Alzheimer's Society - A charity that understands all aspects of dementia. As well as providing information and advice, it funds research into better treatments.
Website: https://www.alzheimers.org.uk/

Anaphylaxis UK - Supports people with serious allergic reactions. Provides information, advice and training.
Website: https://www.anaphylaxis.org.uk/

Asthma + Lung UK - A charity looking after people's lungs. Run by The British Lung Foundation.
Website: https://www.asthmaandlung.org.uk/

Bipolar UK - Supporting people in the UK with Bipolar. As well as providing information and advice, it also runs local support groups.
Website: https://www.bipolaruk.org/

Borderline Support UK - A charity supporting people with Borderline Personality Disorders.
Website: https://borderlinesupport.org.uk/

British Heart Foundation - Provides advice and information about all things cardiac.
Website: https://bhf.org.uk/

British National Formulary (BNF) - Provides information about medications that is useful for healthcare professionals prescribing or administering medication.
Website: https://bnf.nice.org.uk/

Cancer Research UK - Provides advice and information about Cancer, also funds research into better treatments.
Website: https://www.cancerresearchuk.org/

Cardiac Risk in the Young - A charity that provides information for those that have lost someone to Sudden Cardiac Death.
Website: https://www.c-r-y.org.uk/

Crohn's & Colitis UK - A national charity providing information, support and funding research for Crohn's & Colitis in the UK.
Website: https://crohnsandcolitis.org.uk/

Cystic Fibrosis Trust - Provides advice and information for people living with Cystic Fibrosis.
Website: https://www.cysticfibrosis.org.uk/

Diabetes UK - A charity that provides valuable information for people living with all forms of diabetes.
Website: https://www.diabetes.org.uk/

Elton John AIDS Foundation - A charity that aims to prevent HIV infections, educate and inform, provide care for and reduce stigma for people living with HIV across the world.
Website: https://www.eltonjohnaidsfoundation.org/

Endometriosis UK - A UK charity providing information, advice and support for women affected by Endometriosis.
Website: https://www.endometriosis-uk.org/

Epilepsy Action - Provides advice and information about epilepsy.
Website: https://www.epilepsy.org.uk/

Family Planning Association - Provides information around contraceptive methods, although a lot of their leaflets and resources have an associated cost.

Website: https://www.fpa.org.uk/

Fibromyalgia Action UK - A national charity providing information and support for people with fibromyalgia in the UK.
Website: https://www.fmauk.org/

FSRH UK - The Faculty of Sexual and Reproductive Health (FSRH) UK provides guidelines on the issuing of Emergency Contraception and Contraceptive Methods in the UK.
Website: https://www.fsrh.org/home/

General Medical Council (GMC) - The independent regulator of all doctors in the UK.
Website: https://www.gmc-uk.org/

JDRF - A Type 1 Diabetes charity that funds research into a cure and better treatments for people with Type 1 Diabetes.
Website: https://jdrf.org.uk/

Kidney Research UK - A national charity providing information, advice and funding into Kidney Research.
Website: https://www.kidneyresearchuk.org/

Lupus UK - A national charity that provides support for people living with Lupus in the UK.
Website: https://lupusuk.org.uk/

Macmillan Cancer Support - Provides advice, information and support to people living with Cancer.
Website: https://www.macmillan.org.uk/

MIND - A mental health charity delivering advice, information and support.
Website: https://www.mind.org.uk/

Motor Neuron Disease Association - A national charity providing support around Motor Neuron Disease and funding research into the disease.
Website: https://www.mndassociation.org/

MS-UK - A charity that provides advice and information about MS.
Website: https://ms-uk.org/

Muscular Dystrophy UK - A national charity that provides a variety of information for people with Muscular Dystrophy and funds research into better treatments.
Websites: https://www.musculardystrophyuk.org/

National AIDS Trust - A charity that educates around HIV/AIDS and is responsible for the Red Ribbon campaign.
Website: https://www.nat.org.uk/

National Institute for Clinical Excellence (NICE) - Guidelines for best evidence-based practice in the UK.
Website: https://www.nice.org.uk/guidance

NHS Inform (Scotland) - The National Health Service (NHS) is the UK's healthcare provider organisation. NHS Inform is Scotland's website for health information.
Website: https://www.nhsinform.scot/

NHS Website - The National Health Service (NHS) is the UK's healthcare provider organisation. Their website contains a wide range of information including: information on conditions, treatments and how to access healthcare in the UK.
Website: https://www.nhs.uk/

NSPCC - A national children's charity that among other things runs ChildLine.
Website: https://www.nspcc.org.uk/

Nursing & Midwifery Council (NMC) - The independent regulator of Nurses, Midwives and Nurse Associates in the UK.
Website: https://www.nmc.org.uk/

Parkinson's UK - A charity that provides information and funds research around Parkinson's in the UK.
Website: https://www.parkinsons.org.uk/

Patient - A useful website providing a wide range of information and tools about health and healthcare.
Website: https://patient.info/

Pulmonary Hypertension Association UK - Provides information and funding for research into better treatments for people with Pulmonary Hypertension.
Website: https://www.phauk.org/

Relate - Provide couples counselling across the UK.
Website: https://www.relate.org.uk/

Re-Solv - A national charity that provides information and advice around use of glues, gases and aerosols. Including the risk of instant death on every occasion of use.
Website: https://www.re-solv.org/

Resuscitation Council UK - Provides guidelines around resuscitation in the UK.
Website: https://www.resus.org.uk/

Royal Osteoporosis Society - A national charity advocating for better bone health.
Website: https://theros.org.uk/

SADS UK - A charity providing information around SADS and prevention (such as defibrillators).
Website: https://www.sadsuk.org.uk/

Sleep Apnoea Trust - Provides support to individuals who experience sleep apnoea.
Website: https://sleep-apnoea-trust.org/

Stroke Association - Provides support for people that have had a Stroke.
Website: https://www.stroke.org.uk/

Terrence Higgins Trust - A UK charity supporting people living with HIV.
Website: https://www.tht.org.uk/

The British Skin Foundation - A charity that funds research into a range of skin conditions.
Website: https://www.britishskinfoundation.org.uk/

The Thalassaemia Society - A national charity that provides information and resources around living with Thalassaemia.
Website: https://ukts.org/

The UK Sepsis Trust - A charity aiming to reduce preventable sepsis-related deaths.
Website: https://sepsistrust.org/

Joke: How do you hide a £10 note from a Surgeon?
Put it with the patient's observation charts.

Afterword

Over the past two decades the focus has been on better treatments for diseases. This is most likely because medical research is often funded by big pharmaceutical companies that make their money from selling medicines to treat long term conditions and diseases. But better symptom management and preventing further damage caused by diseases shouldn't be the aims of medical research.

The aims of medical research should be:

1. To understand the exact cause of diseases/conditions.

2. To develop cures where possible that as a minimum prevent further damage, but ideally reverse the damage and allow the body to heal itself.

It is my sincere hope that over the next two decades, these become the aims of medical research and that we make good progress in achieving these aims.

Healthcare professionals do an incredible job and are often referred to as Heros, at least in UK society. How amazing would it be if patients and their relatives were greeted by Healthcare professionals that could offer cures, rather than limited treatments? This is the sort of world I want to live in.

So take this book as it is, the best cures and treatments at time of publication. I hope that in the future this book becomes so outdated due to the amount of new cures and treatments that I have to remove it from sale.

My Very Best Wishes,

Antony Simpson - Registered Nurse

Wednesday 20th March 2024

Joke: Why did the Nurse need a red crayon?
Because she needed to draw blood.

Index